Cancer Caregivers

A Resource Guide

Hundreds of Essential Tips

Karen Kirzner Adler

Rozlyn Forman Kleiman
MEd, MA, ATR

General Disclaimer

This book is designed for personal information and educational purposes only.
It is not engaged or intended to render medical advice or professional services.
It should not be used in place of appropriate medical treatment from a qualified
medical professional.

The contents of certain material presented is constantly changing; every effort
has been made regarding the accuracy or currency of the information at time
of printing.

Caregiver Information

If found, please return...

Name:

____

Address:

____

____

____

E-mail:

____

Phone:

____

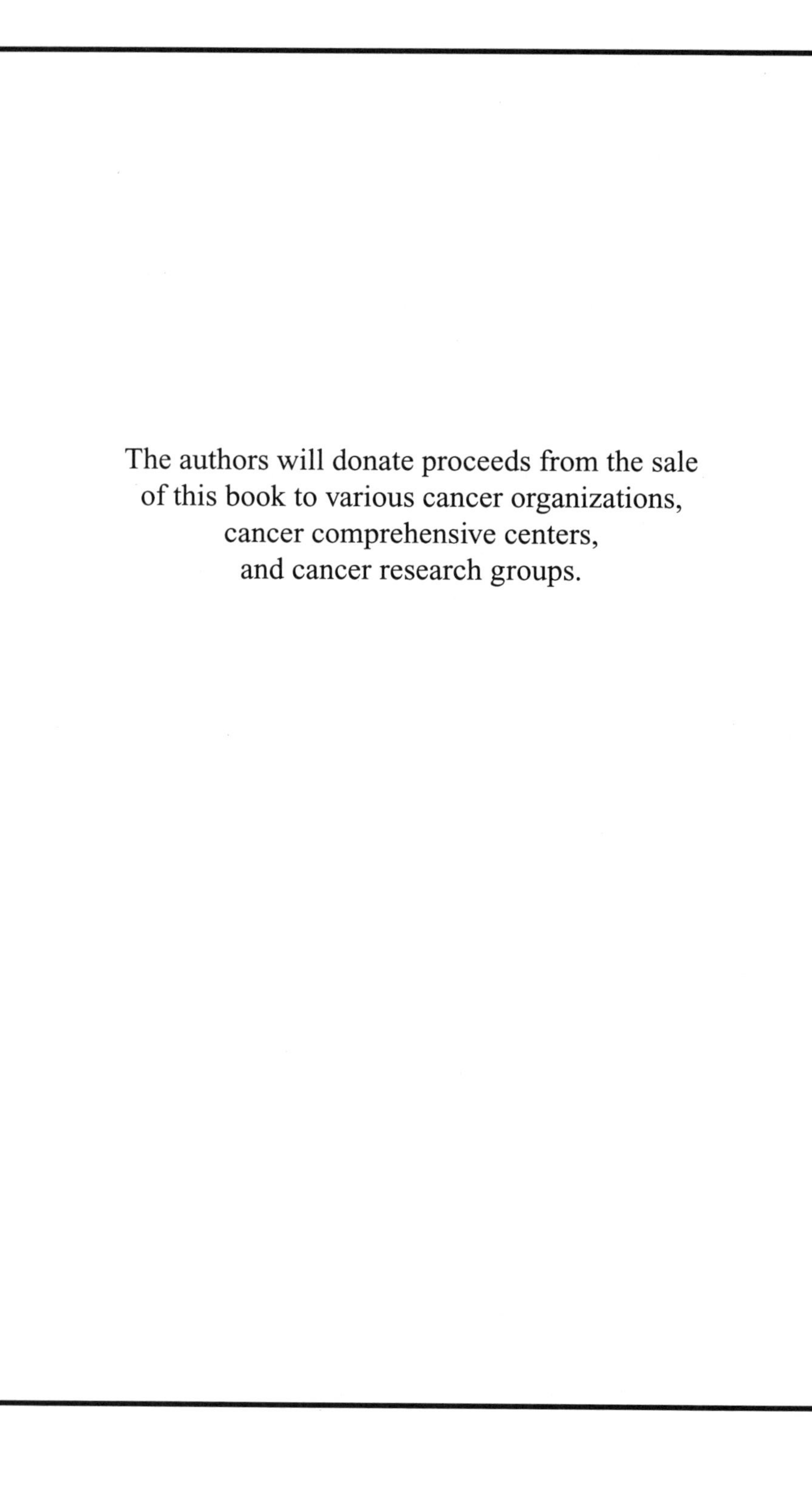

The authors will donate proceeds from the sale
of this book to various cancer organizations,
cancer comprehensive centers,
and cancer research groups.

We dedicate this book to
our loving husbands
whose fight for survival
became our fight.

To
Monty, who lost his battle
on June 27, 1997
and
Marty, a survivor.

Contents

Contents

Contents

Acknowledgments

Monty and Karen wish to acknowledge the following persons:

Dr. Ellie Goldstein, my cousin, who guided us from the start. Not only did he direct us to the best doctors and help us interpret medical information, he also reassured us, and was simply a true friend.

Dr. Melani Shaum, Monty's oncologist, kept us calm and always on the right track. Her knowledge, compassion, patience, and availability were extremely comforting throughout Monty's illness. Dr. Shaum's nursing staff, especially Kimberly, took wonderful care of Monty. A very special thanks to Jenny for her efficiency and her caring attitude that kept me at ease. She was always willing to put me in touch with Dr. Shaum or to help me figure out what to do.

Dr. Jeffrey Hagen, Monty's surgeon at USC University Hospital, who followed Monty's progress throughout his illness. Dr. Hagen's confident attitude kept us calm through extremely difficult surgeries. Also many thanks to his nurses, Leslie and Patsy, who were always "on call" for assistance or reassurance.

To friends and family, especially the Kirzners; mom and dad (Bessie and Joe), Jeff and Christi, Eddie, Phyllis, Sid and Nehama Adler, Monty's son, Josh, Laurel Nathanson, Stu and Joan Lenoff. We don't know what we would have done without your love and support.

Marty and Roz wish to acknowledge the following persons:

Dr. Philomena McAndrew, Marty's oncologist, who was "on call" day and night and insisted that we forge ahead with treatment, despite opposition and warnings from her medical team. The Cedars-Sinai medical staff, including the bone marrow transplant team; the nursing staff at Cedars-Sinai. Of special note, the seventh and eighth floor nursing staff whose support and accommodations went beyond nursing. Also, the seventh floor physical therapists who, upon Roz's recommendation, insisted Marty get out of bed whether he wanted to or not. Without their insistence, he would still be in bed. The blood facility team who gently took blood and platelets from us on a weekly basis. To the associates of the department, Dr. Sam Pepkowitz and Dr. Ellen Klapper, who sat numerous times answering questions and discussing theories with Roz.

Dr. Rick Sokolov who saved Marty's life more than once. Marty gave him the opportunity to become an expert on every unusual infectious disease known to man. Dr. Clive Segil, orthopedist, operated on Marty more than 27 times. He made Marty a new man. His artwork is displayed on Marty's body. Dr. Levi Meier, Cedars-Sinai chaplain, continues to help us emotionally and spiritually. Every encounter adds new light, encouragement, and hope. One's life is enhanced by crossing his path.

To our family and friends, too numerous to individually mention, your constant visits and phone calls have continuously encouraged and positively supported us. A thank you is inadequate; our hearts are overwhelmed and full knowing you are part of our lives. To Pam and Sheri, Roz's daughters, a special note of love for their consistent support and positive spirit. To Marty's children for being there for their father.

An acknowledgment from Monty, Marty, Karen, and Roz to:

All the other physicians, nurses, and home health care professionals who made life calmer, easier, and more hopeful.

Your emotional support is our crutch. Without your love and support this path would be very tedious and difficult.

We are fortunate, to have *all* of you in our lives.

What Cancer Cannot Do

It cannot cripple love

It cannot shatter hope

It cannot corrode faith

It cannot eat away peace

It cannot destroy confidence

It cannot kill friendship

It cannot shut out memories

It cannot silence courage

It cannot invade the soul

It cannot reduce eternal life

It cannot quench the spirit

—Anonymous

Introduction

When illness occurs to someone close to us, we want them to have all the comforts and quality of life that we can help provide. People live with illness longer as advances in medical science increase. A person is more apt to recover when attended to by a loved one; thus enters the role of the "caring" caregiver.

From our experience as caregivers, we have learned and collected many useful tips and essential functions that we would like to share with you. This book is a result of our collection of hundreds of personal notes and tips from our journals, extensive research on cancer, and caregiving. We structured the book by providing practical, ready-to-use tips on the right-hand pages. We share our many caregiving experiences in short vignettes on the left-hand pages.

One way to alleviate negativity is to express it, expel it, and then get rid of it. In each section of this book, we give you this opportunity by providing a space for your personal thoughts. Use these spaces to journal your own thoughts and feelings, questions, conversations with physicians, and any other information you need to express and record.

Whether you are beginning your journey, in the midst of the journey or just know someone else who is, we hope that you will find this book a great comfort and a valuable tool as you take on the responsibility of providing "caring" care for the cancer patient in your life.

—Karen and Roz

Becoming Caregivers

Sometimes when people meet, an immediate bond forms and a meaningful, lifelong friendship develops. This is what happened with our group of six teachers from Emanuel Day School in Los Angeles. During the early 1980s, we formed a camaraderie that lasted beyond our individual departures from Emanuel. To this day, we meet for dinner once a month.

During the last 17 years, all of us have experienced changes within our families. Over the years, we have shared laughter and tears, marriages, births, illness, and death. At our monthly dinners, we share and receive comfort, solace, advice, and friendship from one another. We tried to extend our mutual devotion, entanglement, and involvement to include our significant others. But the few times spouses were included, our conversations were filtered, strained, and less intimate. We decided to keep it "girls night out."

The men had little in common. Sadly, it took an illness to bring Karen and Roz's spouses together. In May of 1995, Monty and Marty found a common thread. Monty was diagnosed with esophageal cancer at USC University Hospital and Marty had a hip replacement—*on the same weekend.* Marty continued to suffer and two months later at Cedars-Sinai, he was diagnosed with multiple myeloma. The men spent the next two years consulting and consoling each other as they tried to conquer this insidious disease. Monty would describe his latest find on the Internet and Marty would expound on his life's philosophy of "things happen" (only much more profoundly). They kept each other's spirits up when they wavered.

Monty's diagnosis of esophageal cancer (Stage III) was a shock. He appeared to be in excellent health and had no history of any illness. Cancer was not an expected path in his life. Monty's battle began with a 12-hour surgery. After recovering from surgery,

Monty was told that he would face an uphill struggle "because survival of esophageal cancer at his stage was uncertain."

He was told that he had 6-12 months to live. With this information, we began the bumpy, uphill road that other cancer patients and their loved ones have faced. Monty was determined not to let this disease get the best of him. Even after surgeries and different chemotherapy treatments, Monty always continued to investigate new treatments. He continued to live his life to the fullest. He took advantage of every moment and every day.

As a mathematician, he often calculated the statistics of various treatments. He always maintained that he would beat the odds. Monty spent numerous hours doing research on the Internet, in medical libraries, and calling cancer centers around the world. Throughout his illness, he displayed a tremendous amount of strength, courage, and determination. He maintained his sense of humor, positive spirit, and attitude. Although Monty gave a courageous fight, his battle was lost on June 27, 1997.

A few words that describe **Marty** are tenacity, stubbornness, persistence—all wrapped around a unique sense of humor. Although you can take the boy out of Brooklyn, you can't take the Brooklyn out of the boy! Marty transplanted with his family to Los Angeles in the 1940s. He entered the "Big One," World War II, where he received a Purple Heart. After the war, he became a business entrepreneur and the owner of various businesses.

The qualities that made him a success in business transferred over to his journey with cancer. Marty, the patient, inspired his doctors. Beyond medical reasoning, doctors pursued treatments not usually administered to a 68-year-old man. Marty underwent an autologous transplant (bone marrow transplant using his own stem cells).

Marty also had a clean bill of health. Marty's plight began the day after Mother's Day in 1995. He complained of immense leg pain which led to 17 surgeries, including a hip replacement and removal of his fourth lumbar vertebrae.

During the following months, Marty's weight dropped from 235 pounds to 145 pounds. We knew something wasn't right. We were persistent with the doctors and demanded that they keep looking, however, they could not pinpoint the problem. It wasn't until the middle of July when an oncologist finally diagnosed Marty as having multiple myeloma. We were told that a bone marrow transplant was the only hope of survival. Marty, who loves to gamble, encouraged doctors to "play the odds." From June 16 until December 26 our home became Cedars-Sinai Medical Center in Los Angeles.

Marty underwent multiple surgeries, chemotherapy, bone marrow transplant, infections, intensive care units, and continuous movement from room to room and floor to floor. (The only floors he missed were the maternity and children's wings!) He had two code blues (cardiac pulmonary arrest). In 1996, he returned to the hospital on a monthly basis for one infection or surgery after another. The years following have been more tranquil, although Marty is still occasionally admitted for an operation or an infection.

He has monthly bone strengthening treatments and, as of today, his cancer is in remission. We constantly research new treatments and discoveries and are willing to try what is available. Marty has resumed playing golf. As an avid golfer, Marty's golfing drive is what keeps his aim high and positive.

In addition to our regular jobs, caregiving to our husbands became our vocation. We were able to support each other by discussing what was happening in our lives, choices we would never make again given the same set of circumstances, and sharing strategies and ideas for making daily life easier to cope. We hope this book makes it easier for you to cope throughout your own journey.

1

Beginning
A Whole New World

In the Beginning

Diagnosis

*You are about to embark on a new path where
enlightenment will ease the journey.*

Beginning Questions to Ask

- Is the tumor benign or malignant (cancerous)?

  ____

- What type of cancer?

  ____

- Where is the site of origin?

  ____

- If malignant, has it spread (metastasized)?

  ____

- What are the options for treatment?

  ____

- Will this treatment cure the disease or merely palliate it?

  ____

- What is the most aggressive course of action?

  ____

To request information about the patient's specific cancer,
contact:

800-ACS-2345 (800-227-2345)
American Cancer Society
www.cancer.org

800-4-Cancer (800-422-6237)
National Cancer Institute
Cancer Information Service
www.nci.nih.gov

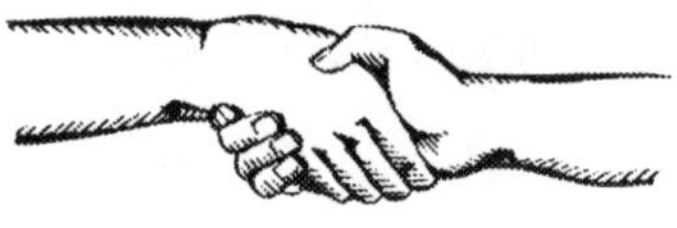

Never give up on anybody. Miracles happen every day.

—*H. Jackson Brown, Jr.*
Life's Little Instruction Book

Personal Thoughts

____
____
____
____
____
____
____
____
____
____
____
____
____
____
____
____
____
____
____

Selecting Oncologists, Surgeons, Physicians and More Physicians

Interview and get more than one opinion before you select your physicians. No one will become closer to you on this journey. Trust will become the most important factor in your search for a physician—listen to your instincts when evaluating a doctor.

What Questions Do You Ask the Oncologist?

Prepare questions prior to doctor's appointment. This list of questions is by no means exhaustive.

- Are you a specialist in this type of cancer?

- How many patients have you treated with this specific cancer?

- Can you provide us (patient and caregiver) with references of other cancer patients? *Call them.*

- Do you work with a partner or a team?

- Will the partner/team "step in" when the primary doctor is not available? *Be introduced to partners (write their names down).*

Personal Thoughts

- Is there always someone on-call (24 hours, 7 days, and holidays)?

- Will you communicate and coordinate with other specialists (surgeon, internist, radiologist, etc.) concerning the patient's progress? *It is important to have every doctor involved with the patient's progress.*

- Is there someone in the office always available to provide test results?

- Are you opposed to using state-of-the-art procedures or new research?

- Are you opposed to the patient trying alternative medicine (see page 113) as an adjuvant therapy in addition to conventional medicine?

- Will you support the patient if he/she wants to try new alternatives?

What Questions Do You Ask if Surgery is Required?

- How many operations of this type have you performed?

- Can you predict the successfulness of the operation?

- What is the usual ratio of success?

- What are the risks?

Personal Thoughts

- Can we meet with the anesthesiologist?
  (Write down name.)

____

If you are comfortable with the anesthesiologist, continue to request her/him for all surgeries.

Adjuvant Treatment

Adjuvant or auxiliary treatment is added to increase the effectiveness of a primary therapy such as surgery or radiation.

- Will adjuvant therapy (see Glossary) be needed?

  ____

- What follow-up treatment will be required, such as chemotherapy or radiation?

  ____

- How often will the treatment be required?

  ____

- Will there be any side effects? What are they?

  ____

- If there are side effects, do we call the doctor immediately or wait until the next visit?

  ____

- What, if anything, will be needed?

  ____

- What are the newest medications to combat side effects?

  ____

- Besides conventional medical treatment, are there alternative methods available?

  ____

Monty's and Marty's oncologists were always available to communicate with Karen and Roz.

Dr. Melani Shaum was such a caring physician, not only for Monty but for Karen, too. Knowing that Karen was busy caring for Monty during the day, she would call Karen in the evening. The two could leisurely discuss problems, questions, and review Monty's progress without interruption.

Dr. Philomena McAndrew would come into Marty's hospital room after 9:00 P.M. almost every night. She would discuss all available options, procedures, and prognosis, plus she would discuss personal situations. If Philomena was away during one of Marty's difficult times, she would telephone to see how he was doing.

The devotion, affection, and commitment these doctors have for their patients give the families the courage to fight this disease.

— Roz and Karen

If at any time the patient or caregiver is not comfortable with the doctor, you have the right to choose another doctor.

Rapport is critical, especially as time goes on.

Pertinent Suggestions

- Contact a prominent medical school near you and speak with the Oncology Department chairperson for research information and doctor referral.

- Consider a doctor and a hospital within close proximity to the patient's home.

- Consider a doctor and hospital which uses state-of-the-art methods.

- Ask how you can receive the latest information on new research and medication.

- Advise your doctor that the patient is willing (if true) to try any new/trial procedures. You as caregiver are willing to be supportive.

- Schedule patient's appointments to coordinate with your daily routine, if possible.

- Schedule first/early morning or late afternoon appointments, so you won't have to spend the entire day waiting at the office.

- If an appointment is in the afternoon, call to confirm appointment and ask if doctor is on schedule.

- If you work, schedule treatment appointments toward the end of the week, so you can be home on the weekend with the patient.

- Befriend the doctor's nurses; they are a good source for information.

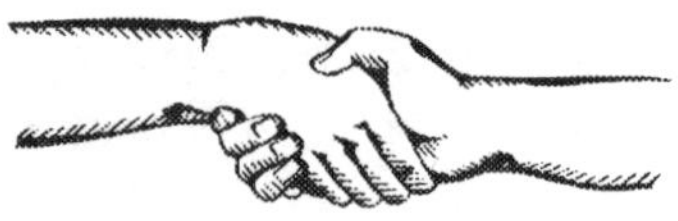

Monty's favorite outing was stopping for ice cream on the way to his doctor appointment. This became a ritual. We looked forward to sitting outside, talking, and enjoying the moment.

— Karen

Marty and I always scheduled afternoon appointments for his chemotherapy treatments. On his treatment days, we had a ritual: Marty would go to work in the morning and then meet me for lunch. After lunch, we would rent a video to watch at the doctor's office while Marty received his treatment. We incorporated cancer into our way of life.

— Roz

Personal Thoughts

____
____
____
____
____
____
____
____
____

- Booklets/pamphlets are found in the hospital/ oncologist's office. Take advantage and read them.

- Ask the doctor's office if they validate parking. If not, ask if there is a monthly or reduced rate available. Parking can be expensive, especially while having chemotherapy treatments and other lengthy appointments.

- You and the patient should take reading material, knitting, etc. to the doctor's office. Waiting can be more productive and less tedious if you are engaged in an activity that is fun and familiar to you.

Personal Thoughts

Consulting with Your New Friend, the Oncologist

If you are accompanying the patient to his/her doctor's appointment, include a pleasant activity before or after the visit.

Things to Do

- See a movie
- Go to a museum
- Go to a park or a zoo
- Walk around a mall
- Eat in a restaurant
- Go to a coffee house, ice-cream parlor, etc.

What Are Some Possible Concerns?

To prevent the "I should have asked" syndrome, make a checklist of items to ask the doctor and bring it with you to the appointment.

- What medications, vitamins, or herbs should the patient take?

  ____

- What new medications are available?

  ____

- What are the upcoming tests or previous test results?

  ____

Personal Thoughts

- What new research information is available?

  ____

- Does insurance cover each and every new procedure?

  ____

- What are the side effects?

  ____

- What is the worst case scenario?

  ____

- What is the name of person(s) to call in case of emergency?

  ____

- Which appointments can the patient go to alone (if they are able)?

  ____

- Which visits require the caregiver's presence?

  ____

- If the caregiver cannot stay for the entire treatment, can the patient be accompanied to the car or lobby by an attendant or nurse?

  ____

- What activities can be continued or discontinued?

  ____

- What type of exercise can be done or should be avoided?

  ____

- Regarding the immune system, should crowds be avoided?

  ____

- Are there any dietary restrictions?

  ____

Personal Thoughts

Remember to

- Ask the doctor about *all* new information or procedures.
- Bring all new research and clinical trial data that you have found.
- Bring questions that you and the patient have prepared prior to the appointment.

Tips

- Always allow patient to make choices and final decisions.
- During regular treatment/routine visits, let patient go to the appointment alone, if possible. However, advise the doctor beforehand in case new/pertinent information is discussed and your presence is needed.
- Often times another person is needed to help take in and decipher information that the patient is too mentally or physically overwhelmed to comprehend.
- Remember that the patient needs to maintain independence. The patient can lose hope and become despondent if he/she feels overly dependent upon others and out of control.
- Encourage the patient to play an active part in life and in information gathering. It is easy to become complacent.
- *Always* respect the patient's wishes and requests.
- *Remember you are a caregiver, not a controller.*
- *The patient needs to be in control of his/her illness and his/her recovery.*

Keep the patient empowered.

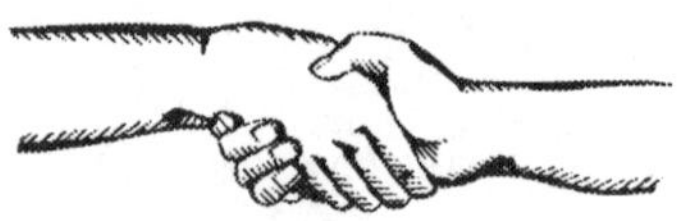

Monty's friends and family donated blood for his surgery. Getting involved was important for them and Monty felt confident receiving this blood.

— Karen

I kept a list of people who were able to donate blood and those who also had matching blood type. Our friends, Brian and Kelly, who had the same blood type, always donated when it was an emergency.

Marty constantly needed platelets and blood transfusions. Often our kids and I would donate blood or platelets whenever we could.

— Roz

We followed up with thank-you notes.

Personal Thoughts

____
____
____
____
____
____
____
____
____

Blood Donations

Donor centers are located in local hospitals or a local community blood center such as the American Red Cross. When blood or platelets are necessary, these facilities are very helpful.

What Should You Know About Giving Blood or Platelets?

- Hospitals will provide blood. There could be a charge for special handling of directed donations.
- Appointments can be scheduled for blood donations, however, platelet donations must be scheduled.
- Ask if there are any specific requirements for donation.
- You cannot give blood if you:
    - take certain medications
    - have a cold or have had certain illnesses
    - have traveled to a malaria-prone country within the last year

Ask friends and family to donate blood, especially those within a reasonable distance of the hospital. People often are willing to help. Keep a list of names, addresses, phone numbers, and blood types for future use. Send a thank-you note to each person after they have donated.

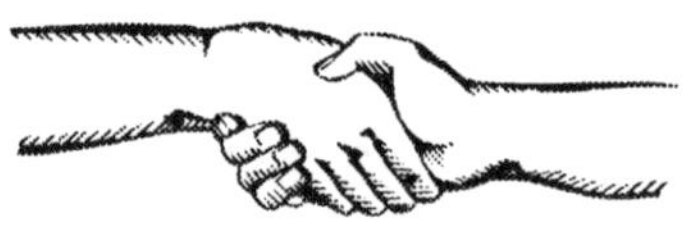

The machine for platelets is amazing to see. It takes a few hours to give platelets. The donor is connected to the machine with a needle in each arm. The machine separates and collects the platelets. You need to squeeze a ball to keep the blood flowing.

Some hospitals have a special machine for platelet donations needing only a one-arm hookup. This machine takes a little bit longer but it allows you to have one hand available to read a book or scratch your nose. Ask for this when you make your platelet donation.

If the hospital donor center is closed on the weekend, you can donate at the nearest Red Cross and they will transport the blood/platelets to the hospital.

— Roz

Personal Thoughts

Giving Blood

- Blood needs to be compatible with the patient.
- Blood can be stored for 42 days following donation.
- Blood takes 45 minutes to donate, from start to finish.
- Whole blood can be donated once every eight weeks.

Giving Platelets

- Platelets do not have the same compatibility requirements.
- Anyone can donate platelets.
- Platelets must be used within five days of donation.
- Platelets take three hours to donate, from start to finish.

What Should You Know About Blood Count Results (CBC)?

These are usual (norm) CBC results.

- Blood counts list the number of platelets and white and red blood cells in a sample of blood.
- Red blood cells are part of the blood that brings oxygen to the tissues and takes carbon dioxide away from them.
- Hemoglobin (iron-containing, protein-carrying oxygen) and hematocrit (percentage of blood volume) are the tests used to evaluate the red blood cells.
- White blood cells are part of the blood that helps fight infection within the body.
- The immune system is affected if the white count is above or below the normal range (4K–10K/ul).
- Platelets are a part of the blood that helps clotting.
- A normal platelet count range is between 150K–400K/ul.

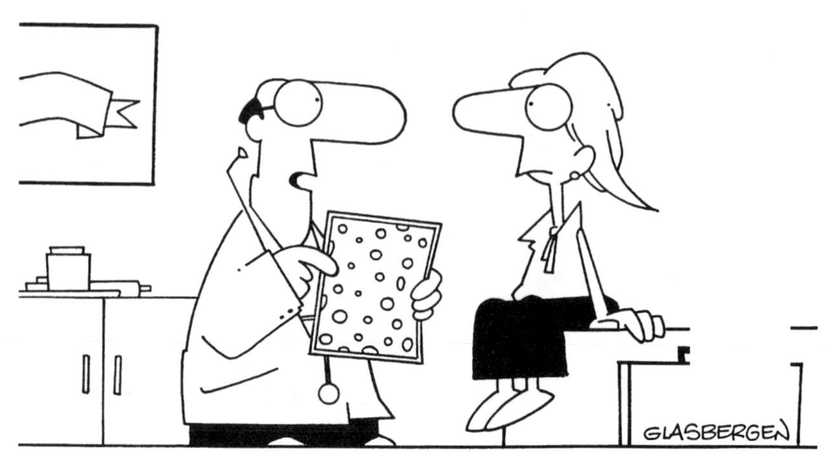

**"The red blobs are your red blood cells.
The white blobs are your white blood cells.
The brown blobs are coffee. We need to talk."**

Personal Thoughts

- Each time blood is drawn, ask for a copy of the patient's blood count.
- Each individual's disease may cause blood results to vary.
- Consider charting the patient's counts.

Tips

Obtain the maximum amount of blood that the patient might need. Unused blood will be donated and used for others. Make sure people at the blood bank credit the patient's account in case of future needs.

Sometimes the hospital donor center hours are not convenient. In that case, the local community blood center will deliver donated blood to the hospital. Check with your local blood center for any restrictions.

To find a local American Red Cross chapter, contact:

American Red Cross
800-448-3543
www.redcross.org
(enter your zip code for a local agency)

If you ever have extra time while at the hospital, donate blood or platelets. The hospital always needs extra blood and platelets. They will be very appreciative.

Get to know the people who work in the blood unit.
They will be there for you.

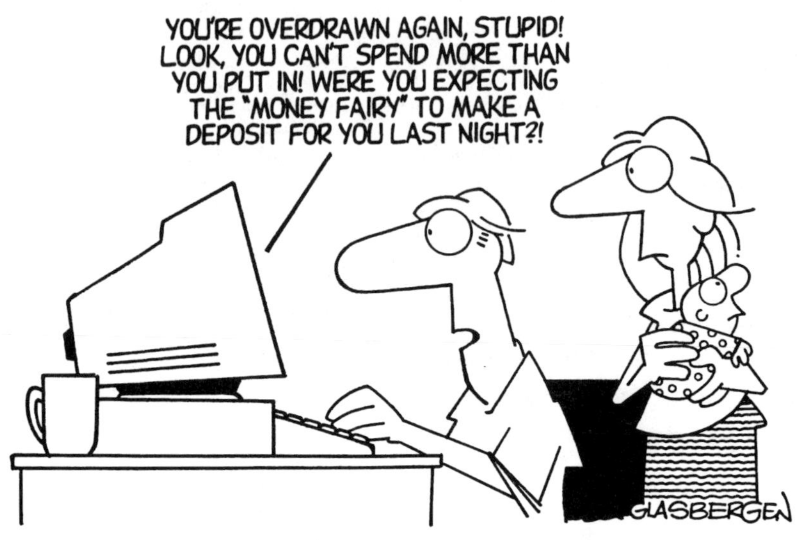

"I liked our old accounting software better."

Personal Thoughts

Directory of Professionals

Keep a list of professionals used by the patient or professionals the patient intends to use in the future.

Who Are These Professionals?

- Accountant

  ____

- Attorney

  ____

- Banker

  ____

- Doctors

  ____

  ____

- Hospital

  ____

- Chaplain

  ____

- Social Worker/Counselor

  ____

- Support group leader

  ____

- Financial Representatives

  ____

- Insurance Agents

  ____

- Real Estate Agents

  ____

Each name and phone number should be easily accessible.

You need to keep copies.

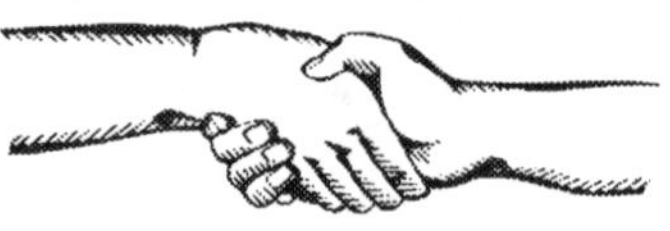

A journey of a thousand miles begins with a single step.

—*Confucius*

Personal Thoughts

____
____
____
____
____
____
____
____
____
____
____
____
____
____
____
____
____
____
____
____
____

Who's Who

In each doctor's office, medical service center, and hospital, you will meet people whom you will see regularly throughout your journey.

Helpful Hints

- Get to know office staff. They will become responsive to your needs.
- Get to know the nurses, receptionists, and the entire staff.
- Always greet them by name and with a smile.
- Be sincere and show interest in them.
- Bring small gifts of appreciation for the office such as candy or cookies.
- Remember them at holiday time.
- When calling the doctor's office, speak with the nurses you and the patient are familiar with and who know your case history.
- Only call them when it is a true emergency.
- Sometimes you can speak with the physician's nurse or assistant (PA) instead of the doctor. If not, leave a message for the doctor to return your call when it is convenient.

Remember these people are very compassionate, otherwise they would not be in this profession.

Show your appreciation.

2

During

And Enduring

HOSPITAL

It is important to feel comfortable in the hospital surroundings. Hold onto the positive attitude and hope that this stay will improve the patient's status.

Throughout your journey, you and your loved one will travel back and forth to the hospital. Stays may last for a few days or a few weeks. It is important to learn your way around the hospital so that you can feel at ease.

What Would Make You More Comfortable?

Get to know the hospital staff:

- Social Worker

  ____

- Chaplain

  ____

- Head nurse for every shift

  ____

- All room nurses and aides

  ____

- Interns/Residents

  ____

- Dietitian/Nutritionist

  ____

- Volunteers

  ____

- Person in charge of parking/parking attendants

  ____

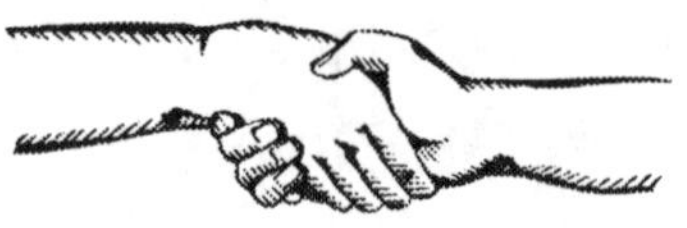

Our time at the hospital was, on the whole, without incident. When a problem did occur, it was usually resolved by a head nurse, who are wonderfully efficient. Occasionally, negative situations occur but if you act promptly, you can rectify the situation.

One time, Marty had a high fever and was bleeding. He needed to transfer to ICU. Being a weekend, the nursing staff was limited, slow-moving, and attending to other matters. Friends who were visiting us became agitated and began moving Marty's bed themselves. The nurses came running, insisting we were not allowed to move the bed. After a confrontation between our friends and the nurses, Marty's bed was quickly moved to the ICU.

Overall the hospital staff is extremely helpful. When you encounter a nurse who is not courteous, try to understand the tension and pressure of his/her job. If there is an ongoing problem with a particular nurse, speak to the nurse in charge or the social worker.

— Roz

Personal Thoughts

- Cafeteria Workers

____

- Room custodians

____

- Security personnel (especially if you need a late night
escort to your car)

____

Social Worker

The social worker is an excellent source of information.
Besides guiding you to the proper resources, they can help
you in very troubled and problematic times. Inquire about
special rates. Ask if there are in-hospital support/group
services you can attend.

Chaplain

There should be a chaplain and a hospital chapel available.
Seek this out. If one is not available contact your own place
of worship or ask the social worker or head nurse. Visit a
chaplain and develop a rapport. The chaplain is a great
source for strength. The chapel is a marvelous place for
solitude, meditation, and some private moments to focus
and gain inner peace.

Nurses

By making friends with the head nurse on every shift, you
will be able to receive the status information concerning the
patient. You may also get "off-the-cuff" advice and
information, but you *must* ask for it. Approach the head nurse
by asking, "What have you seen . . . ?" or "From your
experience . . . ." Inquire about "off-the-cuff" alternative or
auxiliary services/treatment. Wait for the appropriate time to
approach the nurses when you need information.

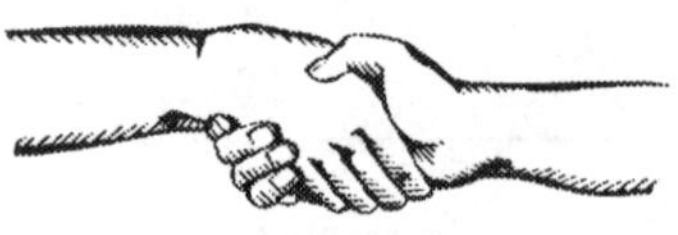

Marty was in the hospital starting in May 1995 for approximately 250 days. Parking at the hospital cost $10 per day. It would have cost me, out of pocket, $2,500 plus doctor appointments. Our children were at the hospital continuously. Adding their cost to mine would have cost over $12,500. This is just for parking; therefore, parking arrangements are necessary.

— Roz

Personal Thoughts

Be courteous to all of the nurses; learn when you can approach them and when it is not a good time. Never approach during shift changes or meal time.

Bring gifts of appreciation for the entire floor, such as candy or cookies. Also, bring a package labeled specifically for the "Night Shift." When the patient is discharged from the hospital, leave flowers or candy that the patient received for the nurses. They love and deserve it.

Get the phone number of the nurses' station desk so you can call 24 hours a day to get information about the patient.

Always leave your home, work, or cell phone number with the nurse in case of an emergency.

Volunteer Hospital Group

Visit the volunteer office. Inquire about services they provide and how they may help in your individual situation.

Dietitian/Nutritionist

The dietitian/nutritionist can assist you with the patient's dietary needs or preferences. Find out if you can bring in ethnic food. Obtain permission for all incoming food as the patient may need a restricted diet. If permission is granted, ask a nurse to note this on the kardex (a small card placed on the front cover of each patient's medical file). The dietitian/nutritionist can also allow you kitchen access and provide you with extra snacks.

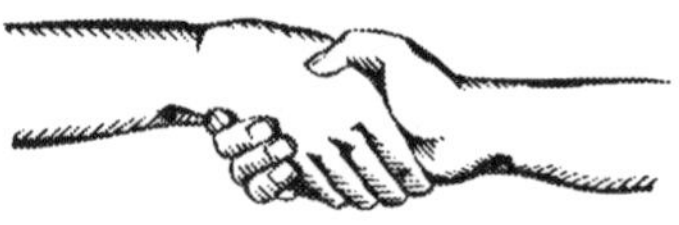

As we shared this experience, we learned that life is a journey with many roads. You may encounter many obstacles and detours. Sometimes the trail that you are following seems endless, but it will eventually lead to another. Hold on to the vision, concept, and faith that eventually you will reach a smoother route. This will give you the strength and coping ability to face each day. Always keep this within you.

— Karen and Roz

Personal Thoughts

Parking

Most hospitals charge for parking. Often times the hospital has special weekly and monthly parking rates. Discounted prices may be available for senior citizens, financial hardship, or other special cases. You *must* inquire. You can find out about rates from the parking office, hospital administrator, social worker, or chaplain.

If needed, ask the social worker if the hospital offers paid taxi service and have the social worker arrange this service. If the doctor's office is part of the hospital, inquire about discounted parking passes when patient is receiving treatment at the hospital.

Hospital Cafeteria/Meals

If you are constantly visiting or staying at the hospital, find out if there are discounted prices offered in the cafeteria or dining room. Verify cafeteria hours. Reduced hours may occur during weekends.

Ordering in food is fun and a change for both you and the patient. Nurses have take-out menus and restaurant delivery information and can usually tell you which restaurants deliver the best food. When ordering, ask the nurses if they want anything.

Hospital Amenities

The hospital is like any other corporation; they want your doctor's business and yours so they offer certain frills. What special amenities does your hospital offer? The social worker can give you many of the answers. Many of these amenities are not in the room; ask about them. The TV usually has a directory of hospital services and amenities. Refer to the proper channel.

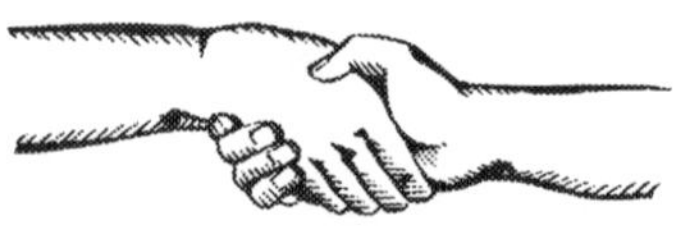

Learn to listen. Opportunity sometimes knocks very softly.

—*H. Jackson Brown, Jr.*
Life's Little Instruction Book

Personal Thoughts

____
____
____
____
____
____
____
____
____
____
____
____
____
____
____
____
____
____

Possible Amenities

- VCR
- Movies/informative tapes
- Newspaper/magazine/book delivery (Ask Volunteer Services)
- Refrigerator in the room

    Often times, a small refrigerator can be placed in the room.

    If not, find out where you can use one.
- Meals for the caregiver
- Cots
- Shower available for caregiver
- Overnight caregiver/family accommodations

If there is a cost for an amenity, you or the patient will be responsible. Insurance will not cover costs or reimburse you.

Hotel

If the hospital is a distance from your home, find out if there is a nearby hotel. Ask if the hospital offers any special rates or extended stay discounts. Call the American Cancer Society for information on discounted rates. Contact the National Association of Hospital Hospitality Houses, Inc. at 800-542-9730 or the Ronald McDonald House at 630-623-7048.

Education

- Take advantage of the education, support groups, and lectures at the hospital.
- The hospital may provide classes, lectures, and television shows on specific topics.
- Does the hospital have a library?

When Marty was in the hospital for long periods of time, I would take up residency there, too. I settled in by having a cot and refrigerator delivered to the room. We kept the refrigerator filled with fruit and goodies. We made it a pleasurable time for us and our visitors. All cards and letters were hung around the room. We ordered in dinners from local restaurants and friends joined us for some evening meals. At holiday time, my sister-in-law brought a home-cooked meal, and we set up a holiday table. I brought my clothes and cosmetics for daily changes. I also brought our mail, paperwork, and laptop computer to the hospital (a computer can be rented on a daily basis).

— Roz

Personal Thoughts

- Is the hospital a designated National Cancer Institute (NCI) Comprehensive Cancer Center? (see page 215)

Patient's Room

- If possible, request a room/bed near a window so there is light and a view.
- Try to get a room near the nurses' station.
- Decorate the room with personal items such as pictures or cartoons.
- Hang up get well cards.
- Display flowers. If you have too many, share them with other patients, the children's ward, or give them to the nurses' station.
- Bring an inexpensive clock.
- Bring a tape player for music or book tapes.
- Bring pads, pencils, and magic slate (this saves paper).
- Bring games, puzzles, books, playing cards.

Emergency Time

Have your physician call the ambulance company for you. If you call, you may have trouble being reimbursed from the insurance company.

If you call 911, *they will take you to the nearest hospital.* This may not be the hospital you have always been admitted to nor the one your physician is on staff.

Surgery Time

- Schedule surgery early in the week (Monday or Tuesday) and the first operation of the day whenever possible.

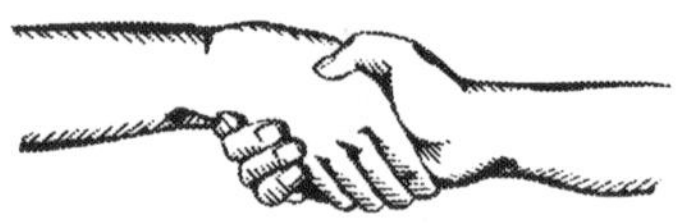

On the day of Monty's surgery, the nurse took our family on a tour of the hospital facilities. The tour included the Intensive Care Unit (ICU) including the room Monty would use after surgery. To help us cope, the nurse explained the ICU rules and identified all of the equipment in the ICU room. Since we learned what the machines and alarms were used for, we did not panic when an alarm went off. We felt more comfortable and knowledgeable about ICU procedures. This information proved helpful and reassuring to our family.

— Karen

Personal Thoughts

- Insist on seeing the patient before surgery. This is extremely reassuring to both the patient and to you.
- Tell surgeon that you will remain in the waiting area on the surgical floor.
- During surgery, remain in the waiting room in case the surgeon needs to do a surgical procedure not expected or any question arises.
- Usually there is a volunteer in the waiting room or a phone number to the surgical unit. Let the volunteer know if you leave the waiting area.
- Leave a phone number where you can be reached or a time when you will return.
- If there is a bulletin board, leave a note.
- Give the waiting room phone number to immediate family and close friends.
- Have your "Sack of Essentials for Everyday." (page 169)
- Following surgery and after speaking to the surgeon, you will be able to leave (if you want to).
- Ask if you can see the patient in the recovery room.
- Patient will be in the recovery room for two to four hours before returning to his/her room — good time for you to take a break!! Take this time to go outside, stretch, and move around.
- Physical activity is a good way to keep your mind clear and focused on the needs of the patient.

Intensive Care Unit (ICU)

Sometimes the patient will go into ICU following surgery or if the patient is medically unstable.

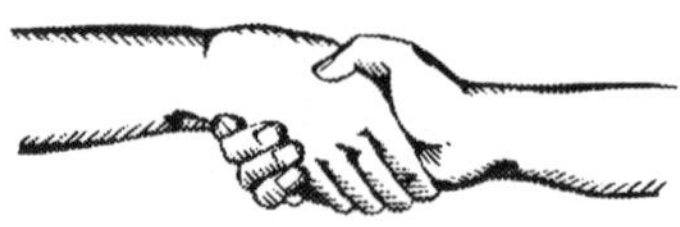

During Marty's stay in ICU there were moments when it was touch and go. One time I was told to make funeral arrangements. My girlfriend Carol went with me to buy a cemetery plot. Marty recovered, and on our first trip out, I took him to the plot site. He was opposed to the location I had chosen. Together we selected another location. This was fine with me because it was less money, and I received a refund.

— Roz

Personal Thoughts

- Get to know the ICU nurses. They are the ones who can and will "bend" the rules. They are very professional and compassionate.
- Ask if nurses are on eight- or 12-hour shift schedules and when they take breaks. *Never* call one hour before or after shift changes.
- Call each morning for a progress report so you needn't rush to the hospital. Take an extra hour for yourself.

The ICU nurse "runs the show."
If you are congenial to them, they may bend the rules.
Always remember to show them your appreciation
and do not take advantage.

- A teaching hospital has interns/residents. They are willing to speak with you at appropriate times.
- Know what time doctors/residents usually make rounds. Be there when you can.
- Know when to stay and know when to leave. Meet the patient's and the unit's needs.
- It is best to leave the ICU when there is a "Code Blue" (cardiac pulmonary arrest).
- When nurses come into the ICU room to attend to the patient, especially in an emergency situation, you must leave.
- Many times you can stay in the room if you are quiet and do not get in the way. Ask the ICU nurse.
- Do not allow more than two people in the room at a time.
- ICU visitation is restricted to close friends and immediate family during scheduled hours.
- Do not congregate in the ICU unit. Use the ICU waiting room.

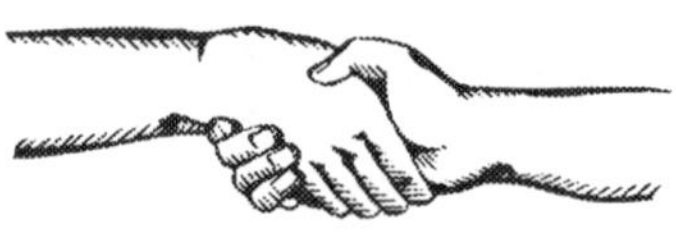

If we were at the hospital when a medication or IV was being administered, we would check with the nurse that it was the correct medicine or IV. If the medication looked different or came at an unusual time, we asked to see the change in the order.

— Karen and Roz

Personal Thoughts

____

____

____

____

____

____

____

____

____

____

____

____

____

____

____

____

____

- Let the nurses know that you are in the waiting room or that you are going home.
- Post your home/cell/beeper phone numbers on the wall of the patient's ICU room.
- Check that nurses write these phone numbers on the kardex.
- Inform nurses who and what information they should divulge to others.
- One person should be the intermediary for patient update. Place that name on the kardex.
- Ask for the direct phone number to the nurses' station.
- A television or music/relaxation tapes are important items to keep the hearing/visual senses functioning. You may need to insist that visual or hearing equipment is allowed in the patient's room.

As caregiver, your goal is to help create positive energy and feedback for your loved one.

The patient is the focal point!

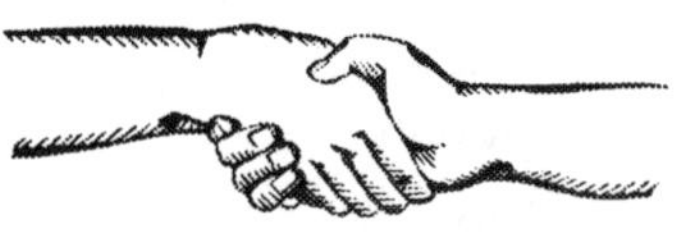

I count myself in nothing else so happy
As in soul remembering my good Friends.

—Shakespeare
Richard II, Act II, sc. 3

Personal Thoughts

Visitors

Some patients thrive on constant visitation from certain visitors, other patients prefer limited visitation, and still others prefer selected visitors. Be aware of the patient's wants and needs during his/her hospital stay.

Advice for Hospital Visits

- Visitors must maintain a positive attitude without placating the patient.

    Inform the visitor of patient's health status and appearance *prior* to the visit. This way the visitor can prepare for a change in the patient's appearance and also maintain or regain a positive attitude.

- Set up a visitation schedule, dependent upon treatments, tests, and patient's capacity to endure.

- Stagger visitors so there are not too many visitors at the same time or on the same day.

- Occasionally ask friends or family to spend a day at the hospital and substitute for you. Select someone the patient is at ease with and does not feel the need to entertain.

- Visits should be short (30 to 60 minutes).

- Keep conversations "normal." Topics of conversation should be those that were discussed prior to patient's illness: everyday chitchat, fashion, business, world events, stock market, sports, etc.

- Be a good listener; the patient may want to vent . . . listen, don't advise.

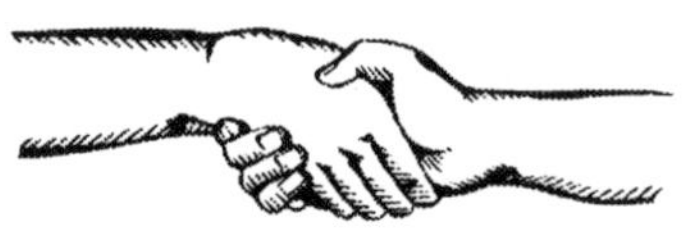

Never deprive someone of hope; it may be all they have.

—H. Jackson Brown, Jr.
Life's Little Instruction Book

Personal Thoughts

- If the patient tells you something in confidence, respect his/her wishes.
- Understand, at times, the patient is sedated/medicated and may appear confused.
- Understand the patient may be expressing wishes rather than reality.

What Some Visitors Might Say or Do When Visiting the Patient

- What is your prognosis?
- How long did the doctor give you to live?
- What did the doctor say?
- What medicines are you taking?
- I have a friend or relative who knows someone who has cancer and you know what happened to them...?
- Refer to the patient in the past tense.
- Recap entire relationship with the patient as if preparing a eulogy. Remember, cancer is not necessarily a death sentence.
- Talk about the patient as if he/she is not in the room.
- Turn to someone else in the room and say, "Tell him/her that..." The cancer does not affect hearing.
- Tell the patient that he/she is not looking well.
- Look shocked at the first sight of the patient's appearance. Remember the patient is very aware of nonverbal signs.

This is not the time for family members or friends to make amends with the patient. If such a visit is requested, ask the patient first, before the visit takes place. The patient's wishes *must be* respected.

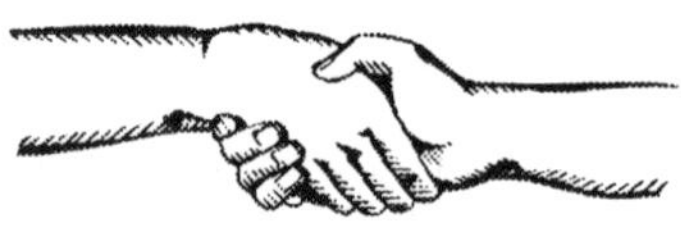

Marty is a born salesman — a real "people" person. He thrived on having visitors. If he was alone, he would sleep to pass the time. I put a sign on the door saying, "OK to wake." He enjoyed conversing and telling jokes. Marty was upset if people came to visit but did not wake him up.

— Roz

Monty enjoyed visits from friends and family but there were times when he needed or desired to rest quietly. It became my responsibility to inform people when Monty did not wish to be disturbed by visitors or phone calls.

— Karen

Personal Thoughts

During a hospital stay, the patient needs to concentrate on his/her wellness and recovery.

What You Should Do for the Patient's Comfort

- While in the hospital, patients sleep at all hours. Ask the patient if phone calls or visits will be disruptive.
- Limit phone conversations — keep them short.
- Turn off the ringer on the phone when the patient is sleeping or resting.
- If patient receives many "drop by" visitors, post a sign on the door advising of the patient's needs.
- Change the sign according to the patient's condition. For example, the sign might read:

  "No visitors at this time."

  "All visitors must wash hands before entering."

  "Please wear a mask."

  "Please limit your visits to xx minutes."

  "Do not enter if you have a cold."

  "OK to wake patient."
  "Check with nurse before entering."

Suggested Items for Visitors to Bring

- Food items adhering to dietary restrictions
- Audio tapes: relaxation, positive readings, humorous tapes
- Movie tapes (if VCR is available)

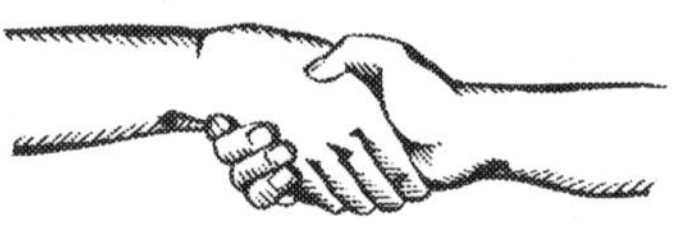

To have a friend you must be a friend. Fortunately, we — Monty, Karen, Marty, and Roz — were very wealthy in this respect. Distance does not matter in friendship. We received constant phone calls from friends and relatives all over the world. To this day, Marty receives a daily phone call from one of his oldest and dearest friends, Jimmy, who lives in New York. We continue to update and visit with our friends through e-mail.

— Karen and Roz

Personal Thoughts

- Books: best sellers, comedy, jokes, crossword puzzles
- Magazines, newspapers
- Radio or tape player with headphones
- Balloons, plants, flowers
- Flowers, plants, fresh fruits and vegetables are not permitted when the white blood count is low after chemotherapy or in patients with leukemia.

Some patients want visitors and others may not. Understand the desires of the patient and proceed accordingly.

Remind visitors how important their visit is to the patient and he/she looks forward to it. This will put the visitor at ease and they will concentrate more on the person than on their own feelings or the cancer.

Ground rules will vary according to the patient's requirements, endurance, and the doctor's orders.

As caregiver, you are in the position to inform friends and family of the patient's current situation.

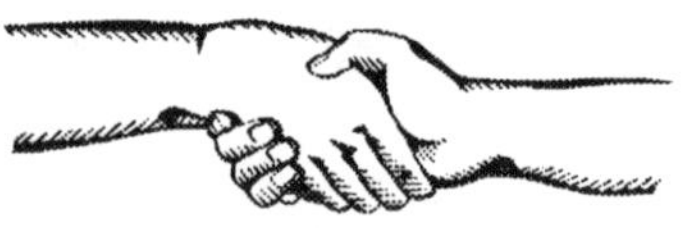

Never waste an opportunity to tell someone you love them.

—H. Jackson Brown, Jr.
Life's Little Instruction Book

Personal Thoughts

Communicating to Others

*Friends and family want and need updated information
especially after surgery or test results.*

How to Keep Everyone Informed

Constant calling and receiving of telephone calls can become exhausting.

- Establish a telephone tree where friends call each other. This will save you time, energy, and hours of repetition.
- Update your answering machine daily with patient information, adding appreciation for the call and forgiveness if you don't respond immediately.
- Use e-mail; you can notify several people at once.
- Indicate if visitors are welcome and best time of day to visit.

*It's important to let people know
how much you appreciate their calls
but
not always to expect a return call.*

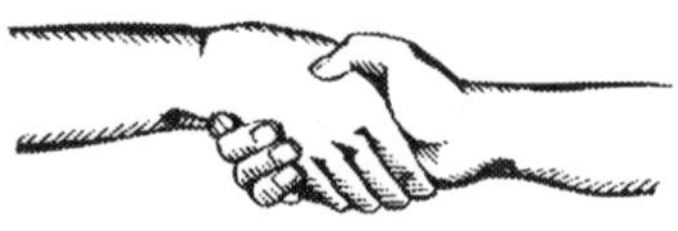

Marty was admitted to Cedars-Sinai Medical Center every few months after his diagnosis. If friends called our house and didn't find us home, they immediately called the hospital. There was a period of time when we considered calling the hospital to retrieve our phone messages.

— Roz

Personal Thoughts

Hospital and More Hospital

If you are in a situation where the hospital becomes an ongoing experience, certain tips can make it a little easier.

What Should You Pack?

- Medical history cards, insurance cards, special instructions.
- A list of all medications the patient is taking, including the dosages and time of day administered. Also list any allergies.
- Comfort items: razor, deodorant, other necessary toiletries (these are not reimbursable from insurance company).
- Pajamas/nightgown.
- Bathrobe and slippers.
- Reading material.
- Glasses, if needed.
- Small currency.
- Phone numbers.
- Pen, note pads, paper, writing journal.
- Inexpensive watch/clock.
- Any miscellaneous "to do" items.

Label everything with the patient's name.

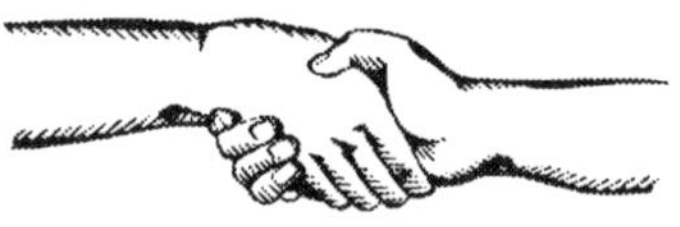

In three words, I can sum
up everything I've learned
about life. *It goes on.*
Despite our fears and worries
life continues.

—*Robert Frost*

Personal Thoughts

____

____

____

____

____

____

____

____

____

____

____

____

____

____

____

____

What You Should Not Pack

- Do not pack anything that will be missed if lost or misplaced.
- Jewelry.
- Large denominations of money.
- Expensive lingerie.

Leave the patient's suitcase in the car the day of surgery. Bring the suitcase to the hospital when the patient is in his/ her room.

Entering the Hospital

- The hospital should have state-of-the-art diagnostic and treatment technology.
- The hospital should have integrated health care services.
- Verify the insurance coverage for home health care. When the patient is discharged from the hospital, you will not have to deal with last minute arrangements.
- The hospital should have specialized care units.
- Unless it is an emergency, avoid surgical procedures or hospital entry over the weekend. Most likely, your attending physician will not be on call, and usually the hospital staff is limited.
- If there is a medical problem over a weekend, phone your on-call physician to verify that waiting for a regular office appointment is appropriate.
- Monday is usually a busy day at the hospital. Try to schedule hospital entry on a Tuesday.
- The patient should try to be the doctor's first surgical procedure of the day.

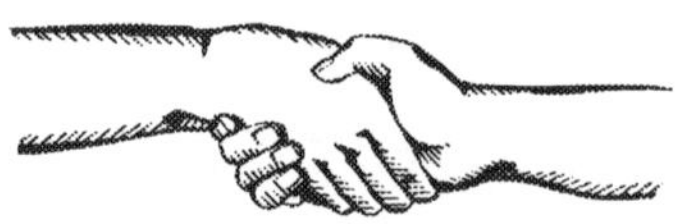

When Marty was in ICU, I insisted that a television be placed in his room when he was awake. Even if he didn't watch it, there was continuous visual and auditory stimulation. I also placed headphones on Marty when he was unconscious and played healing tapes or his favorite music. I asked the maintenance attendant to install an electrical adapter so these accessories would not interfere with the medical equipment.

I believe that visual and auditory stimulation are positive reinforcement healing tools. These tools act as distractors for the patient who is surrounded by disturbing and intimidating machinery.

— Roz

Personal Thoughts

During Hospital Stay

- The best time to ask the hospital nurses for extra help or questions is during their shift, *never* at the beginning or end of the shift or during mealtime.
- Ask if nurses are on eight- or 12-hour shifts.
- Introduce yourself to the nurses in charge of the patient and remember their names.
- Ask for the direct phone line to the nurses' station.
- Ask nurses the appropriate time to phone.
- Always leave the home/cell/beeper phone numbers where you can be reached on the patient's bed.
- Inform the nurses who they can disclose information to and to note it on the chart.
- Ask when the doctor makes rounds. This way, you can be there if you need to speak with the doctor.
- Inquire about visiting hours and rules. Learn how well they are adhered to. Learn which rules can be broken without causing any disruption.
- Keep a change of clothes for yourself in the hospital room.
- Provide the patient with headphones for music and relaxation tapes. Insist that they are allowed, especially in the ICU.
- Let friends and family know if YOU want company during the patient's surgery, if you would prefer being alone, or if you would prefer waiting with only certain people.
- Write in your journal. It may help you to cope with your feelings and release tension.
- Rent or buy books on tape. These are great if you don't want to read.

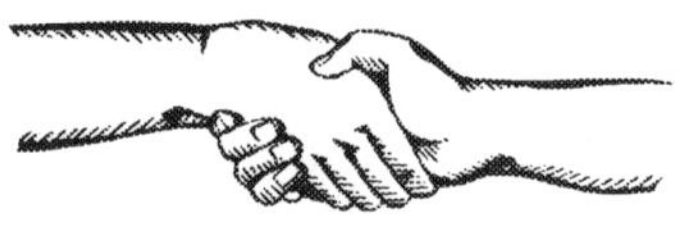

After spending 93 days at the hospital, Marty left on December 26, 1995. Marty's physician, Dr. McAndrew, was out of town. When I asked the nurse to speak with the doctor who prepared Marty's discharge papers, the doctor appeared upset and indicated that the home instructions were with the nurse. He even intimated that I should be grateful that I was even taking Marty home and that I should make him comfortable because, as he said, "there is nothing more to do for him." I immediately phoned a member of Dr. McAndrew's team who met with me and answered all my questions.

— Roz

Personal Thoughts

- Write your phone number on a piece of paper and tape it to the wall near the patient's bed. It will be available, in case of an emergency.

Leaving the Hospital

- Meet discharge nurse or social worker prior to the patient's discharge.
- On the day of discharge (or before, if possible) review the home instruction sheet with the discharge nurse. If necessary, review the instructions line by line and ask any questions while the nurse is available to you and the patient.
- Review the patient's medications and follow-up procedures with the physician and the discharge nurse.
- Have physician or social worker make provisions for home health care, if necessary.
- Prior to discharge, caregiver should prepare the patient's home room to accommodate any special needs.
- Have home health care or medical supply company deliver all equipment to the home at least one day before discharge.
- Check with your insurance company to see what will be covered and how much out-of-pocket cost will be necessary, if any.
- At home arrange for the patient to have close, easy access to the bathroom.
- A day in advance, pick up all medication or equipment from hospital or pharmacy.

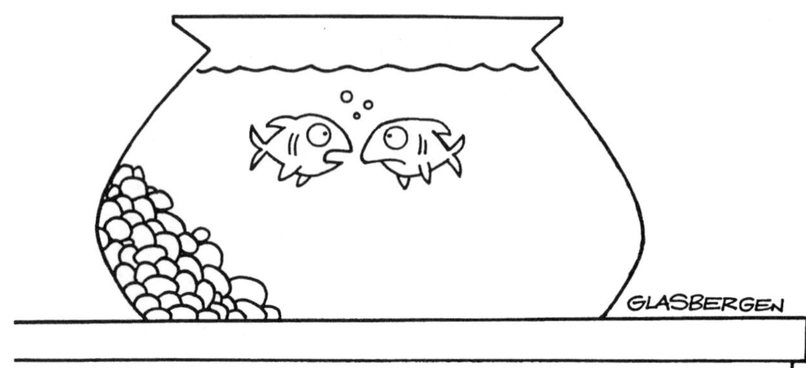

**"I'm leaving you, Gilbert. You can keep
the bowl, but I'm taking the water
and all the colored stones!"**

Personal Thoughts

____

____

____

____

____

____

____

____

____

____

____

____

____

____

____

____

Prescriptions

- Some prescriptions that are prescribed for home use may not be covered by insurance. *Check with your insurance carrier.*
- If you must have prescriptions filled at the hospital pharmacy, ask for a two- or three-day dosage, instead of the full dosage. When you get home, you can compare prices with other discount pharmacies.
- If you decide to get a prescription partially filled, remember to ask the pharmacist to give you the written prescription back as you will need to have it to get the rest of the prescription filled.

What Should You Take When You Leave the Hospital?

Take home all of the supplies from the room as they will come in handy at home. You or the insurance company have already paid for everything, wrapped or unwrapped, that is in the patient's room. If you are unsure as to whether an item is yours or the hospital's, ask the nurse.

- alcohol pads
- clean bedpan
- clean urinals — male or female
- dressing kits
- gauze pads
- small tray
- swab sticks
- tape
- wash basin
- and the *Patient*

Personal Thoughts

Medical Supplies

Assess the needs of the patient! What is needed in the home?

You may not need every item listed below, however, often times, these items are needed initially or are needed for long-term care. By keeping essential items on hand, you will eliminate last minute shopping.

Equipment

Look in the Yellow Pages Directory under Medical Equipment & Supplies *or ask at a local hospital.*

- Bed arm pillow
- Bed liners/bed pads
- Cane
- Chest to keep all medical supplies
- Extra towels, washcloths
- Hospital bed with electrical head and foot components (oversized twin-fitted sheets work best)
- IV pole
- Nightstand with shelves
- Over-the-bed tilt-table tray, bed tray
- Recliner chair
- Shower chair (generally less expensive at a home supply store)
- Shower mat
- Shower/toilet bars installed in the bathroom
- Small baskets to consolidate items
- Toilet seat riser
- Wheelchair

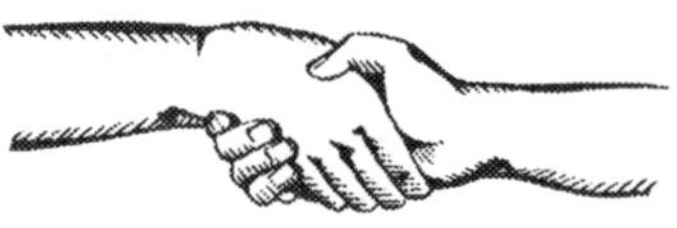

Monty would regularly call the home health delivery service to place his order for medical supplies, which arrived the next day. One time he requested only a few supplies and received a bill for $500. He inquired about the cost and was informed there was a $500 minimum for every order.

We never realized, nor were we ever told, that there was a minimum requirement per order. Had we known, we would have ordered more supplies less often. Once informed of this policy, we immediately changed to a new home health delivery service.

— Karen

Personal Thoughts

What Do You Ask?

- What are the specific insurance company rules regarding equipment?

  ____

- What will the insurance company pay for?

  ____

- Will insurance pay for rental or purchase?

  ____

- If rented, at what point do you own it?

  ____

- What is the minimum and maximum rental period?

  ____

- Is any item more cost-effective to buy?

  ____

- What is tax-deductible?

  ____

Sometimes used equipment is available and is more cost-effective.

Medical Supply Delivery

A medical home delivery service is needed if medical supplies are used on a regular basis (weekly or monthly). Once delivery is established, the company will deliver whether you need the supplies or not.

Check with your home care provider, the oncologist's office, or the hospital if such a service is provided.

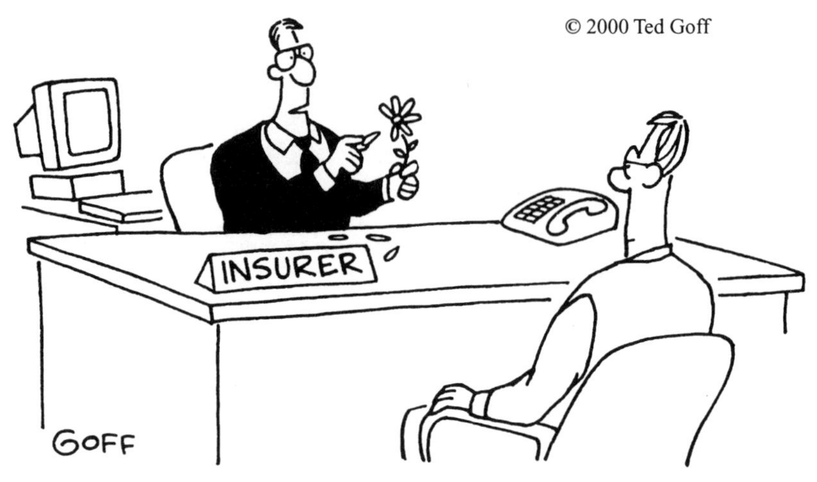

**"We pay you, we pay you not.
We pay you, we pay you not."**

Personal Thoughts

Caution!

- Count your supplies the day before the delivery date—if you have extra items, call and tell them *NOT* to deliver.

- Only get what you really need—excess supplies take up room and you may never use them, as situations change very quickly.

- Excess and unused medical supplies **CANNOT** be returned even if they are in their original unopened packaging—only get what you need.

- When leaving the hospital, check what the doctor ordered for home delivery. Don't duplicate items you already have at home. Take the items from the hospital room that you have paid for.

- If you have home health care, ask the attending nurse to look over the supplies ordered and compare with what you have.

- Many items can be purchased at discount stores.

- Always remember that you may have a cap on your insurance policy. Items add up quickly. Be cautious and selective.

Don't return items that you won't use immediately; you may need them later and then may have to pay another deductible (bed liners, tape, gauze, etc.).

When you are positive these items won't be needed any longer, you can donate them to charity.

I have found through my experience that it is best to make arrangements for home health care through the oncologist's office since that agency stays in contact with the physician and nurses. For example, a relative worked at the first home health care agency that we employed. Naturally we anticipated excellent attention and service. Unfortunately, that was not the case. The agency told our family that there was no reason to administer medicine to prolong Marty's life. They never returned a phone call. Within a week we switched to the agency recommended by the oncologist's office and Marty received excellent care.

— Roz

Personal Thoughts

Home Health Care

As well as having the support of friends and family, a group of professional health providers will ease the task of caregiving.

Often it is necessary to employ a home health care agency when the patient comes home from the hospital or when the patient is very ill. Your oncologist's office or hospital social worker can recommend an agency. The physician must prescribe the need for the service. Policies regarding home health care vary from state to state, so make sure to check with your insurance company and physician.

What Does Home Health Care Consist Of?

- *Nurse*: administers medicine, takes vital signs, and keeps in contact with the doctor.
- *Aide or Attendant*: provides personal care such as bathing, change dressings, change bedding, prepare meals, and clean up for patients.
- *Therapist*: provides physical, speech, occupational, and emotional counseling therapy.
- *Pharmaceutical Needs*: delivers supplies and prescriptions.

Only accept what is needed. Always check with the delivery company to confirm items being delivered prior to delivery. Check with your insurance company as to which supplies and equipment will be covered.

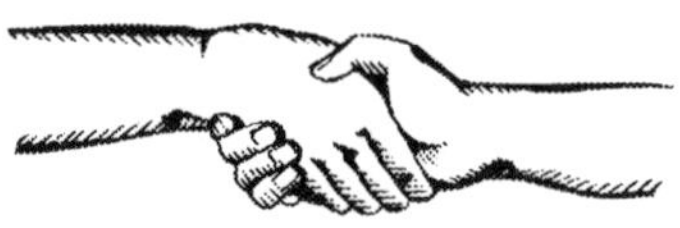

After being discharged from the hospital, Marty was non-ambulatory and confined to a hospital bed for six months. Attendants, nurses, and I cared for him. I kept all supplies easily accessible. I placed a chest in the bathroom for all his medical needs. Near Marty's bed I placed shelves for his personal items, such as daily medicines, papers, books, etc. This kept it simple and organized for everyone.

— Roz

Personal Thoughts

Items to Keep at Home

Select an area in the patient's bathroom where all supplies and equipment will be located. If needed, purchase a small chest with drawer and a cabinet area. This will make it easy for the nurse and attendant to know where everything is located.

Keep these supplies on hand:

- adhesive strips
- antacid
- antibacterial soap
- anti-diarrhea medicine
- body lotion
- cotton balls
- cotton swabs
- cotton swab sticks
- disposable gloves
- gauze pads
- hydrogen peroxide
- iodine swabs
- paper cups
- paper towels
- powder
- rubber bands
- rubbing alcohol
- scissors
- surgical tape
- thermometer
- tissues
- towels
- trash bin
- trays
- tweezers
- urinal/bedpan
- washbasin
- washcloths
- water pitcher
- wipettes

Important Tips

- Before setting up home health care, verify coverage with the patient's health insurance company.
- *Always* ask what out-of-pocket costs are covered for administration of IV and medications.
- Some medications and IVs are only covered by insurance if the patient is in the hospital or if it is administered in the physician's office.
- Certain services and items may not be covered by your insurance or Medicare. It is important to check.

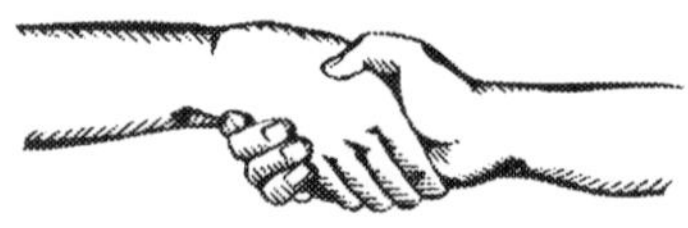

My daughter wrote this during one of my darker moments:

Be Accepting
Be Brave
Be Caring
Be Compassionate
Be Forgiving
Be Loving
Be Optimistic
Be Supportive
Be Sympathetic
Be Tolerant
Be Understanding

JUST
Be There and
Be Together

— Pamela Elyse Sussman

— Roz

- As a caregiver, if you are not comfortable administering or caring for necessary medical procedures, ask the oncologist to prescribe home health care.
- If you are not satisfied with a home health care attendant, ask for a replacement.

If you use an agency recommended by the oncologist,
the agency will be in constant communication
with the doctor's office.

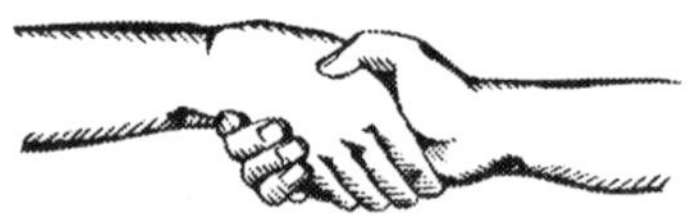

After six months in the hospital, Marty was discharged with a handful of prescriptions. I filled them at the hospital pharmacy and the bill was $2,875. I refused the medicines, knowing that once I accepted them, I could not return them. In a state of shock, I went to the doctor's office to ask which medicines were immediately necessary and which ones were "just in case." The necessary medicines for a few days cost $250.

I decided to pursue other options including Veterans Affairs. Being a disabled veteran, Marty was already in the VA system. Dr. McAndrew helped me make an appointment with the oncologist at the VA hospital. Not only did Marty receive medication for $2 per prescription, but he entered a research program.

— Roz

Personal Thoughts

Medications/Prescriptions

What works when and for what . . .
You are about to learn a whole new world—the world
of prescription and non-prescription drugs.

What About Insurance?

- Many insurance companies offer mail order prescriptions at a reduced rate for long-term medications.
- Generic drugs are less expensive than brand name drugs.
- Inquire from your physician if a generic substitute is permitted for each specific medication.
- Ask your physician or nurse if they have any free samples.
- Contact pharmaceutical companies; they may have programs which provide free prescription drugs.
- Contact the Senate's Special Committee on Aging (202-224-5364) and ask for their free pamphlet "Programs to Help Older Americans Obtain Their Medications" (beneficial for all ages).
- If you are over 50, join AARP because they have pharmaceutical product discounts (800-424-3410).

Insurance policies have various rules regarding pill supplies. If you need a 60-day supply of pills and your insurance coverage only pays for 30 days, ask the physician to write "take as directed" or "take twice a day" instead of "take once a day" on the prescription form. The insurance company will then pick up the cost of the 60 pills.

When you receive the medicine, remember to mark the correct dosage.

What You Should Know About Medications

Ask your physician or pharmacist the following questions:

- Are there any precautions or warnings you should know?

  ____

- Should the patient avoid any foods while taking the medicine?

  ____

- Is it better to take the medication on a full or empty stomach?

  ____

- Is the medicine to alleviate a symptom or to cure?

  ____

- What is the best time of day to take the medication?

  ____

- Can the dosage be altered?

  ____

- If dosage is missed, should patient double up on dosage?

  ____

- Are there potential interactions with other medications, herbs, vitamins, or supplements?

  ____

- What side effects might be experienced?

  ____

- Which side effects need immediate attention?

  ____

- Can the patient abruptly stop the medicine?

  ____

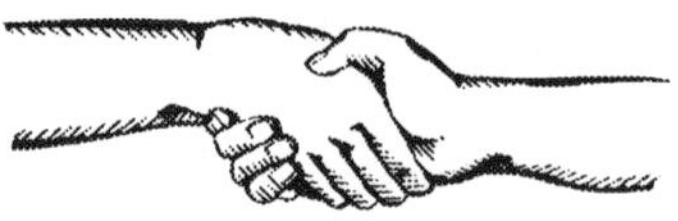

From our experience, we suggest using the same pharmacy and befriending the pharmacist. It is important to notify the pharmacist of all prescription, non-prescription, and alternative medicines that the patient is taking. That way the pharmacist can track and be aware of any drug interactions and side effects. The pharmacist as well as the doctor can advise you regarding drugs that the patient is taking.

— Karen and Roz

Personal Thoughts

____

____

____

____

____

____

____

____

____

____

____

____

____

____

- Are there special storage precautions for the medication?
- Alert your physician and pharmacist to any drug allergies.
- Always inform physician and pharmacist of other drugs patient is taking.
- Ask for a written prescription with the drug brand name and generic name.
- Try to anticipate when the patient will run out of medicine. *Do not wait* until the weekend or evening to call the physician's office for a refill.
- Remember that pain medication alleviates pain. It is advisable to take it prior to any physical activity, if necessary.

What Should You Know About Pharmacies?

- Generally, you cannot order or refill narcotics over the phone. A new prescription must be brought to the pharmacy.
- Ask if the pharmacy offers home delivery service. Find out in advance—it may be needed at a later date.
- Is the pharmacy open 24 hours a day?
- If not, is there another pharmacy nearby that is?
- Have prescriptions filled at an off hour (early morning, dinner hour, or late evening). This will save you time and reduce the chance of a mistake.
- Conduct price comparisons—discount pharmacies vary in prices.
- Request easy-open tops on bottles. Avoid childproof caps, unless you need them, and tell the pharmacist to note this on your record.

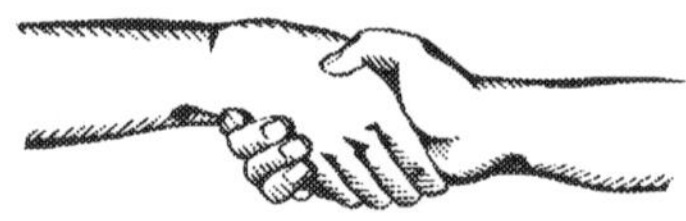

Monty took different medications at various times throughout the day. The number of medications increased as his illness progressed. I found the most organized and easiest way to keep an accurate account was to make a weekly chart. I placed this on the refrigerator door.

Each time Monty received his medication, I recorded it. I put all of the weekly charts in my journal for reference. This was not only helpful to me, but a valuable reference for the doctors and other medical professionals. I always kept an updated copy with me when we traveled.

— Karen

This is a sample of my chart.

Day	Sun	Mon	Tues	Wed	Thurs	Fri	Sat
Date							
Name of Medication							
Time Medication Given							
Dosage/ Amount							
Reaction							

- Ask the price of the medication before you order.
- Ask if medication is covered by insurance.
- Get to know your pharmacist.
- Purchase a pill splitter and weekly/daily pill dispenser.

Tips

- When trying a new medication, only get a small amount. Keep a copy of the prescription. Once you know that the medication is effective, fill the remainder of the prescription.
- Ask if there is a minimum amount of medication that needs to be ordered to meet the prescription filling fee.
- Ask the doctor for free samples.
- Keep the labels from all drug prescriptions *OR* keep documentation of :

  - * dosage/date
  - * drug type
  - * prescription number
  - * prescribing doctor
  - * what it was used for
  - * when taken

- Document all side effects the patient experiences.
- Call the physician immediately if there are any side effects.
- Keep all medications and supplies in one location.
- If needed, purchase a small chest for the medical supplies and items.

Always check the prescription drug before leaving the pharmacy. Once you accept the medicine, you own it!

As Marty recovered from the acute stages of his illness, his prescription medications decreased. Rather than taking them intermittently, he was able to take them all at one time. This included both his prescribed medications from his oncologist and vitamins and herbs prescribed by his holistic physician. (Marty's oncologist recommended a holistic physician.)

Marty began taking all his medications in the morning and would consistently regurgitate. The doctor suggested taking them before breakfast, then after breakfast, then a few at a time but he still couldn't keep them down. Finally one day I suggested he take them at night. This immediately solved the problem. We proved to ourselves how we cannot give up. Keep trying alternative methods with any problems or issues that confront you.

— Roz

Personal Thoughts

Purchase a book on prescription and non-prescription drugs. It will be very informative and also provide information regarding side effects.

Two comprehensive books are:

> *Complete Guide to Prescription*
> *and Non-Prescription Drugs*
> by H. Winter Griffith, MD.
> Berkley Publishing, New Jersey, 1999
>
> *The Pill Book*
> by Harold M. Silverman
> Bantam Publishing, New York, 1998

Other resources can be located in the Cancer Resource Guide in the back of this book.

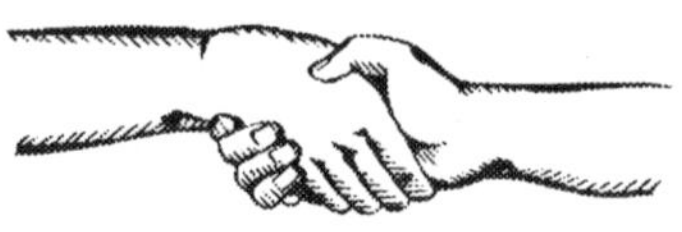

One of the most useful items we had was the disabled parking tag. Wherever we went, we were able to park nearby. This was especially necessary when Monty's energy level was low. Being able to park in front of the theater or a restaurant gave us the opportunity to spontaneously get out of the house, because as Monty would say, "I got to get out into the world!" It made excursions much easier for us.

— Karen

Personal Thoughts

Transportation

Keep a positive attitude by not tracking your miles. Just enjoy the freeways and scenery as you drive.

Pertinent Suggestions

- Contact your local Department of Motor Vehicles (DMV) to apply for a *permanent* or *temporary* handicap tag. The doctor's office may have applications available. A letter from the doctor verifying disability may be required.

- Join an automobile club in case of an emergency. Keep the card handy—one copy in the car and one copy in your wallet.

- If buying a new car, consider one which is easy and appropriate for the patient's needs. Will the patient be able to get in and out of the car easily? Will a wheelchair readily fit?

- Consider purchasing a cellular or digital telephone for emergency situations.

Keep an Emergency Bag in Your Car

The bag should include:

- adhesive strips
- antacid
- antibiotic ointment
- anti-diarrhea medicine
- change of clothing
- medical insurance cards
- pain reliever, non-aspirin
- paper towels
- rubbing alcohol
- scissors

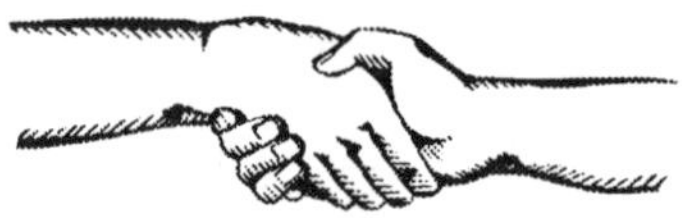

During the time Marty was non-ambulatory, he was transported by ambulance to and from the physician's office for chemotherapy treatment. I received bills from the ambulance company indicating the insurance company paid for the arrival to the physician's office but not the return ride home. This situation is frustrating and defies logic. The hassle continues between the ambulance, insurance companies, and me.

— Roz

Personal Thoughts

- cotton swabs
- cotton swab sticks
- disposable gloves
- doctor names, phone numbers
- emergency medications
- hydrogen peroxide
- trash bags
- thermometer
- towel
- washcloth
- water bottle
- wipettes

- and any special needs of patient

Transportation to Medical Appointments

Sometimes you are unable to accompany the patient to an appointment.

Try these options:

- Some hospitals provide transportation service.
- American Cancer Society has volunteers who drive.
- Check local organizations for volunteers.
- Check universities or high schools for a student who needs to earn extra money.
- An ambulance may be able to transport, especially if patient is non-ambulatory. Check your insurance coverage.
- Some religious groups provide transportation.
- Refer to "What can friends and family do" section of this book.
- Many taxi companies provide special discount rates for this type of transportation.
- Check small van transportation companies.
- Check, if applicable, senior citizen discount rates.

One night I dreamed I was walking along the beach with God. Many scenes from life flashed before me. Sometimes there were two sets of footprints, other times there was only one.

I noted that during the low periods in my life, when I was suffering from anguish, sorrow or defeat, I could see only one set of footprints, so I said to God:

"You promised me, God, that, if I followed you, you would walk with me always. But I have noticed that during the most trying periods of my life there has been only one set of footprints in the sand. Why, when I have needed you most, have you not been there with me?"

God replied, "During your times of trial and suffering, when you see only one set of footprints, it was then that I carried you."

- Author unknown

Personal Thoughts

____

____

____

____

____

____

____

Radiation Treatments

Radiation therapy is a common method of treating cancer in a localized area.

When is Radiation Used?

- Before surgery to shrink the tumor.
- After surgery to destroy any cancer cells that remain in the localized area.
- To relieve pain.

What Does Radiation Do?

- Radiation uses high-energy rays to kill cancer cells.
- Radiation stops cancer cells from growing and multiplying.
- Radiation is usually given five days a week, lasting between two and eight weeks depending on the part of the body needed to be irradiated. This spreads out the dosage so normal cells can recover.

What are the Possible Side Effects?

• Diarrhea	• Painful Swelling
• Fatigue	• Skin Reactions
• Nausea	• Vomiting

Medication is now available to alleviate specific side effects.

Tips

- Caregiver should accompany patient for the first visit.
- Apply green aloe vera gel (purchased at pharmacy) after each radiation treatment to prevent scarring.

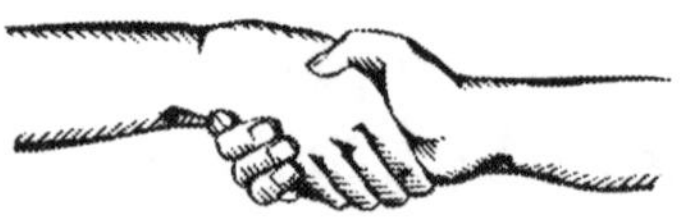

Monty and I conducted extensive research on the Internet and at medical libraries regarding updates and new procedures for esophageal cancer. During his investigation, Monty found a new chemotherapy treatment being implemented at the Royal Marsden Hospital in England. Monty immediately contacted the English researcher and then consulted with Dr. Shaum. The physicians conferred and decided on the best course of treatment for Monty. As a result, Dr. Shaum used this new chemotherapy procedure on Monty.

We were fortunate to have a doctor who was aggressive and open to trying new treatments.

— Karen

Personal Thoughts

Chemotherapy Treatments

Chemotherapy is the use of drugs that are administered intravenously to kill cancer cells.

What Should You Know?

- Various combinations of drugs are used for each individual case. Find out the combination used.

- Chemotherapy is usually administered in the oncologist's office. Length of time varies depending upon combination used.

- Sometimes chemotherapy/radiation can be administered in the hospital or a cancer clinic.

- Schedule treatments when it is the most convenient for you. Usually, a good day is Thursday or Friday, which allows you the weekend for caregiving.

- Some centers offer evening or weekend hours for chemotherapy.

- The patient may be nauseous for 24 hours, however, there is medication available to control the nausea. Ask your doctor for more information.

- One side effect of chemotherapy is hair loss, which can be traumatic. Hats or wigs are often worn. The American Cancer Society issues a catalogue with various hats available to purchase.

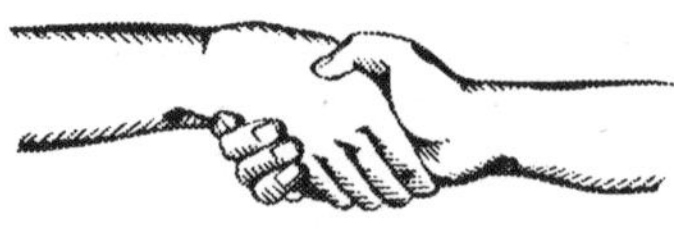

God grant me the serenity
To accept the things I cannot change,
The courage to change the things I can,
And the wisdom to know the difference.

—Serenity Prayer

Personal Thoughts

Tips

- A few days prior to treatment, the patient should begin consuming nutritious meals.
- Encourage the patient to drink lots of fluids.
- If chemotherapy is given in the doctor's office and a VCR is available, bring a humorous video to watch.
- Bring your "Sack of Essentials" (page 169).
- Let visitors know what to expect so they will not be shocked. The patient is very aware of nonverbal signs.

Cancer patients undergoing chemotherapy/radiation and their families can receive information regarding emotional support from:

Cancer Hope Network
Two North Road, Suite A
Chester, NJ 07930
877-HOPE-NET (877-467-3638)
www.cancerhopenetwork.org

*The oncologist's office has information
about the type of drugs being used
for each patient.
Investigate!*

Marty had a stem-cell transplant, and since then his immune system is more susceptible to infection. Marty often needed an antibiotic administered intravenously twice daily. The cost was as high as $600 per day.

Most insurance coverage, including ours, does not include home treatment for this procedure. In order for the insurance company to pay, Marty had to be admitted to the hospital. I questioned and pursued the senselessness of the system to no avail.

— Roz

Personal Thoughts

Immune System

The cancer patient's immune system is in a weakened condition. The presence of the slightest fungus, virus, bacteria, or parasite drains the immune system, making it difficult to fight diseases.

- Ask the doctor about certain vitamins or herbal immune enhancers.
- Be aware of weather conditions and extreme weather changes.
- Patient should dress warmly or carry an extra jacket/sweater.
- Patient should not be around people with colds, especially in confined areas.
- Contact the physician at the first sign of a cold (you or patient), so antibiotics can be prescribed.
- Transmission of germs most often occur through touch.
- Carry a supply of alcohol-based wipettes or antibacterial hand lotion.
- Wash your hands anytime you are doing something for the patient.
- Use plastic gloves when you are treating the patient.
- Patient should have routine checkups with their dentist.
- Patient should try to remain stress-free. Stress accelerates the demands on the immune and endocrine system.
- Thoroughly cook food.
- Refrigerate food immediately.

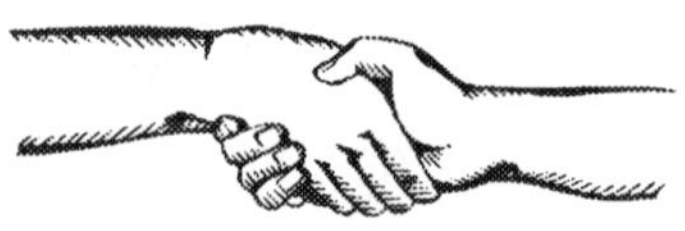

Monty supplemented his diet by drinking a balanced nutritional energy drink, however, he complained about the taste. To make it more palatable, Karen prepared it in a fancy glass with whipped cream (adding more calories), a cherry, and a straw.

Marty also complained about the taste of these particular drinks, so Roz made it more palatable by giving them all away.

— Karen and Roz

Personal Thoughts

The Pyramid of Food

Nutrition

Remember the food group pyramid? If not, now is the time to review it. The cancer patient will experience weight loss and needs easy-to-digest, high-calorie items as well as following good nutritional guidelines.

High Calorie Suggestions

- A nutritionally balanced energy drink
- Nutrition/power bars
- Protein drinks
- Instant breakfast powders
- Supplements added to foods that can be purchased at nutrition centers.

During Treatment Suggestions

- Avoid spicy foods.
- Drink plenty of fluids, especially water.
- Eat energy foods such as carbohydrates.
- Small, frequent, nourishing meals.
- Avoid heavy meals at night.
- Leave a snack next to patient's bed.
- Carry nutritional snacks that do not require refrigeration.
- Prepare and freeze small meal portions so they are readily available.

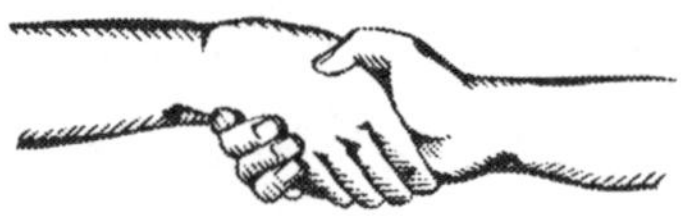

Marty was bedridden for six months. During that time, many friends brought dinner or dessert to our home. I arranged a table in the bedroom and decorated it so that we could all dine together. Even if Marty was having difficulty eating, or did not feel well, our friends visited and we enjoyed each other's company.

Seeing Marty bedridden wasn't easy. We are especially grateful to those special friends who put Marty's enjoyment and happiness first, rather than their own comfort, while sitting through a difficult meal. Marty enjoyed the food and company, and I received a much-needed break from preparing another meal. Those evenings were extremely pleasurable and memorable to us, especially for Marty.

— Roz

Personal Thoughts

General Suggestions

- Often times the patient may become dehydrated; check frequently (ask physician to explain technique).
- Certain sport drinks help restore electrolyte balance and help avoid dehydration.
- Avoid diet drinks and food products.
- Avoid fried foods and refined sugars.
- Check with the physician concerning intake of daily vitamin and mineral supplements.
- Eat one serving of oatmeal per day to reduce fats in the system.
- Limit alcoholic beverages.
- Limit milk and dairy products.
- Reduce fat intake.
- Use lactaid products.
- Eat natural, organic foods.
- Eat an abundance of whole grain products.
- Consider purchasing fresh food products at a natural health food market.
- To coincide with the chemotherapy or radiation treatments ask the registered dietitian or nutritionist to help plan a specific diet.
- Prepare appealing meals by using various colors of food on the same plate.
- If the patient does not feel like eating, do not force food or drink.
- Call physician if patient refuses to eat or drink over a reasonable time period.
- Remember it will be easier for the patient to digest small, frequent meals rather than three large meals per day.
- Keep a list of adverse food reactions.

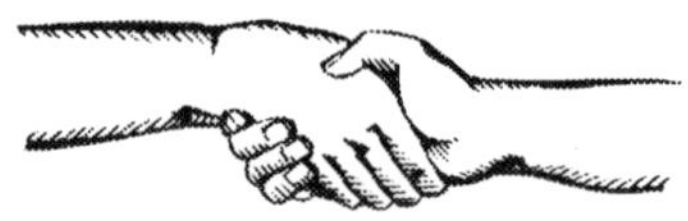

Finding a nutritionist who specializes in cancer patients is important. A qualified nutritionist can prepare a diet according to the specific type of cancer and also prepare dietary guidelines for patients receiving cancer treatment therapies.

During the first phase of chemotherapy, Monty had a difficult time eating. From our research, we realized that food played a significant role in battling cancer and relieving the discomfort during certain or specific treatments. We found a nutritionist who specialized in cancer nutrition. Not only did she introduce us to an overall dietary guide for cancer patients, but she also provided a specific diet for Monty. This included foods to eat and foods to avoid during his chemotherapy treatments. For Monty's specific treatment, he needed to avoid spicy and fried foods and concentrate on eating protein and small, but frequent, meals. He also needed to drink plenty of water in order to remove toxins from his body. By avoiding certain foods and following the nutritionist's recommendations, Monty felt better during his treatments. We found that nutrition was a vital part of dealing with Monty's cancer.

— Karen

Additional Options for Meals

- Community Centers
- Friends/family
- Local Cancer Organizations
- Meals delivered from restaurants
- Meals on Wheels
- Senior Citizen Centers

Registered Dietitian or Nutritionist

- Cancer organizations often have dietitian/nutritionist speakers.
- Ask your oncologist to recommend a registered dietitian or nutritionist.
- Consider consulting with a registered dietitian or nutritionist who specializes in cancer patients to receive proper nutritional guidelines.
- Hospitals usually have a registered dietitian or nutritionist on staff. Call for an appointment.
- Look in bookstores, libraries, and the Internet.

Two informative books are:

5 Minutes to Health by Marilyn Joyce P.O. Box 251300 Los Angeles, CA 90025 310-391-4999 August 1995	*Beating Cancer With Nutrition* by Dr. Patrick Quillin The Nutrition Times Press Tulsa, OK, 1994

After Marty came home from the hospital at the end of 1995, I went to a Chinese herb store and bought the place out! I prepared different teas and gave Marty various herbs that I had heard would help. When he vomited, I didn't know if it was from the stem-cell transplant or from what I was making him. Through the Wellness Community, I was recommended to a nutritionist. Marty was having trouble with his digestive track. He could not keep food down, and for six months, continually vomited and had diarrhea. The nutritionist provided Marty with a specific diet so that he would get the proper nutrients. He had to drink a sport energy drink to keep from getting dehydrated, concentrate on eating a low residue diet, no fruit or vegetable peels, only lactaid milk, plenty of garlic, pasta, tomato sauce, and fish. Anytime he ate something he wasn't supposed to, he would vomit. He still needs to watch what he ingests. Last year he ate oysters and had such a terrible reaction he had to be admitted to the hospital. I soon found out that raw oysters are detrimental to anyone who has an immune system problem or who has cancer.

— Roz

Places to Contact

American Institute for Cancer Research
800-843-8114
www.aicr.org

American Dietetic Association
800-366-1655
www.eatright.org

American Herbalists Guild
435-722-8434
www.healthy.net/herbalists

American Association of Oriental Medicine
610-266-1433
www.aaom.org

Patient should conduct a weekly weigh in.
If necessary, increase food intake.
If a weight loss over 10 pounds occurs,
contact physician.

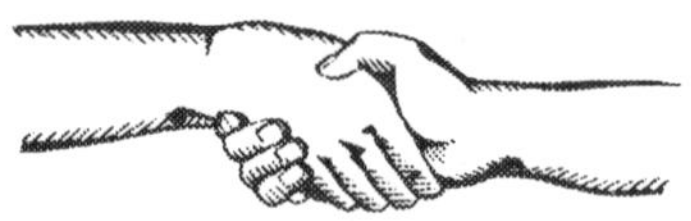

As an art therapist, I am an advocate for alternative medicine/therapy in conjunction with traditional medicine. I had heard of sound therapy. The sound therapist's premise was that sound travels through water quicker than any other matter. Since the body contains 80% water, sound would travel through the body and disrupt the molecules and reorganize them.

One evening shortly after Marty came home from his long hospital stay, I arranged for a sound therapy session; Monty, Karen, and Marty's son Bobby participated. The lights were dimmed, candles were flickering. The therapist began beating his drums and using his special instruments. In the midst of this session, the attending nurse arrived to give Marty his intravenous medication. She entered the room, took one look around, and tore out of the house never to return again.

— Roz

Personal Thoughts

____

____

____

____

____

____

____

____

Complementary and Alternative Medicine

Complementary medicine is non-traditional medicine and is not designed to replace traditional treatments. It can be used in conjunction with mainstream modalities to add a multi-dimensional approach. Alternative medicine has not gone through a rigorous scientific process but is used instead of conventional treatment.

What Does Complementary and Alternative Medicine Include?

- Biological medicine—
    tries to regenerate and correct imbalances in the immune system using various methods including detoxification, oxygen therapy, etc.
- Naturopathic medicine—
    a natural intervention using plant derivatives
- Homeopathic medicine—
    uses vaccines to neutralize the frequency of the abnormal cells so they can no longer function
- Acupuncture
- Cellular Therapy
- Chiropractic
- Hoxsey Therapy—using herbs as an alternative
- Immunotherapy
- Laetrile Therapy

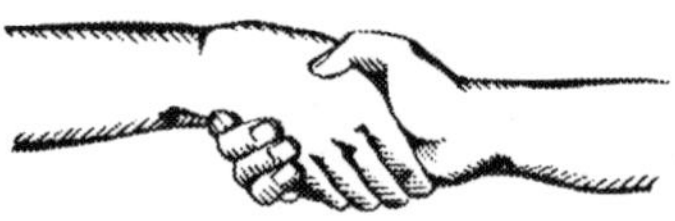

I have always had houseplants to enhance my surroundings. When Marty was in the hospital, I bought plants for his room. I remembered someone telling me that spider plants were particularly good for keeping an area germ free. I hung three spider plants around Marty's hospital room. I always keep an aloe vera plant in case Marty burns or scars himself. He applies the sap to his skin. It promotes the healing.

— Roz

Personal Thoughts

- Macrobiotics—food regimen
- Massage Therapy
- Metabolic Therapy

There are many clinics that offer alternative options. They are costly, however, some insurance companies cover partial cost.

University of Texas—Center for Alternative Medicine
800-392-1611
www.mdacc.sph.uth.tmc.edu/utcam

National Center for Complementary and Alternative Medicine (NCCAM Clearinghouse)
888-644-6226
http://nccam.nih.gov

To receive a complete list of Non-Toxic Therapy and Diagnostic Test directory, contact:

Cancer Control Society
2043 N. Berendo St.
Los Angeles, CA 90027
323-663-7801

Holistic therapy works on the whole body
and mind as a unit.

3

Necessities

Of Life

LEGAL DOCUMENTS

Hope for the best
BUT
Prepare for the worst!

Do not wait until the patient is extremely ill to gather this information. In the event the patient becomes too ill to make decisions, the caregiver must be prepared to take over decision making.

Will

A will is a legal document that names and disperses one's estate upon death. If there is not a will, the state may intercede and probate may be necessary upon death. A will is valid if it is handwritten, not printed or typed.

Durable Power of Attorney

Designates another person to be appointed as a legal representative to manage a person's affairs if he/she becomes incapacitated.

Durable Power of Attorney for Health Care

Designates another person to make life-sustaining decisions on behalf of that person in the event the patient becomes incapacitated.

A document would be given to the doctor and the hospital.

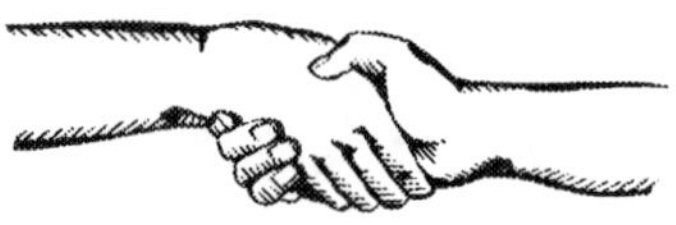

Do not expect family members to respond the way you do; be prepared for anything.

Our experiences included people questioning the will; calling the attorney before the loved one was gone; or insisting the estate be settled immediately after death, prior to any grieving process.

Stay positively focused. Do not allow *your* priorities to become overshadowed by misplaced values.

— *Karen and Roz*

Personal Thoughts

Power of Attorney

Appoints a named individual as an attorney in fact to act in name, place, and stead in any way which the patient would act if he/she were present. The acting person can make financial, property, tax, and business decisions. This needs to be notarized. This does *not* cover medical decisions.

Living Will or Advanced Directive

This is a signed, written statement that informs family members, doctors, and others what the person's preferences are regarding life-sustaining medical procedures.

For more information regarding preparation of living wills and medical powers of attorney for health care, contact:

> *Partnership for Caring*
> *Choice in Dying*
> 1035 30th Street, NW
> Washington, DC 20007
> 202-338-9790
> 800-989-WILL (800-989-9455)
> www.choices.org

> *Place originals in a safe place*
> *and keep several copies*
> *readily accessible.*

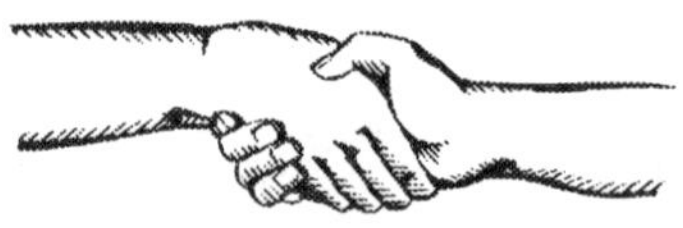

I kept a notebook specifically for insurance information. To keep organized, I divided the notebook into categories. I kept all insurance data, a log of every phone conversation including the date and name of the person I spoke with, payment information, and anything else relating to insurance. This notebook proved to be extremely valuable since I was dealing with the insurance companies on an ongoing basis.

— Karen

Personal Thoughts

Insurance

Keep copies of the insurance card(s) with you at all times.

Those years of premiums are about to pay off! However, you and the patient need to know and understand the coverage. It is estimated that 80 million people have health insurance insufficient to cover the costs of a catastrophic illness such as cancer (Cancer Prevention Alert, 1997).

It is a good idea to contact your insurance agent to review your policy and to find out what is *not* covered as well as what is covered. Find out if you are restricted to certain providers or hospitals (HMO or PPO plans). Retain all policies and addendums. Keep all papers together.

What to Check In the Patient's Policy?

- Maximum and minimum coverage for office visits, drugs, hospital stays, doctor fees, laboratory fees, etc.

- Lifetime maximum coverage?

- Is pre-authorization required for hospital admittance?

- Are emergency admission procedures covered?

- Are ambulance trips covered?

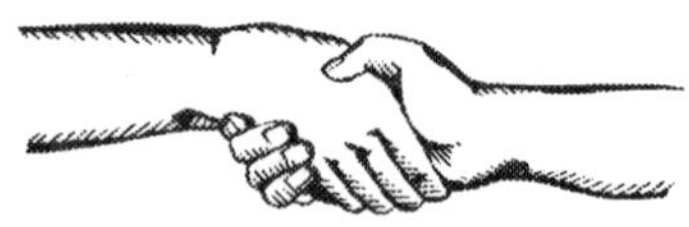

Following Monty's surgery, he needed a supply of catheter dressings. The cost of the first delivery from the home health care provider was $24.95 per dressing. I purchased a similar item at a local medical pharmacy for $7.95 and submitted the bill to my insurance company. They refused to reimburse me even though the price was significantly less. After a thorough investigation, I learned that the insurance company had negotiated with the home health care provider for all purchases.

All future medical supplies needed to be made through the provider if I was to be reimbursed from the insurance company.

— Karen

Personal Thoughts

- Arc laboratory tests and procedures covered?

- Are cosmetic enhancements covered (wigs, hats, bras, etc.)?

- Is emotional support therapy covered? What type?

- Are medical equipment and supplies covered?

- Are prescriptions covered? Which ones?

- Are clinical trials, research and experimental treatments covered?

- Are chemotherapy and radiation covered?

- Are treatments covered in the doctor's office?

- Are treatments covered at home?

- Is hospice care covered?

- Is home health care/home nurse covered?

- Is alternative health care covered?

- Is there coverage if you're out of town or country and immediate/emergency attention is needed?

Personal Thoughts

Insurance companies often require you to submit an authorization letter to release information to someone other than the policyholder. If so, retain a copy for your records.

Always check hospital bills. If additional charges are included, notify the insurance company.

Is the Patient Eligible for Special Programs?

Contacts

- State or local offices to inquire if medical aid or assistance exists.
- Aid to families with dependent children, Social Security office.
- Medical Assistance Programs.
- County Medical Service Programs.
- Greater Avenues for Independence Programs (GAIN).
- In-Home Supportive Services (IHSS).
- Senior Service Programs.
- Social Services within your community, city, or state.
- Supplemental Security Income/State Supplemental Program (SSI).
- Place of worship. They may have an aid program.

Contact your Social Security office, hospital, American Cancer Society (ACS), and local government for information on the above programs.

Having Trouble with Your Claim?

- Ask the insurer why a claim is denied or reimbursed at a lower rate; document the claim representative's name and date/time of call.

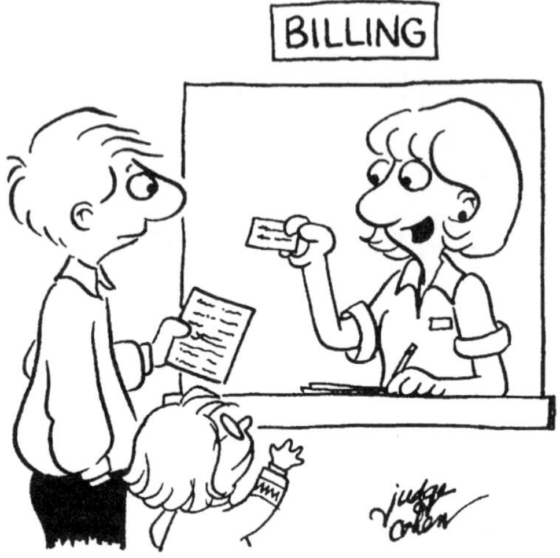

**"Here's the home number for your insurance company's president.
Call him if you have any questions."**

Personal Thoughts

- Contact the billing person at the doctor's office to verify that diagnosis codes are correct.
- Always follow up phone conversations with a letter to all concerned parties (insurance company, hospital, doctor). *Keep a copy.*
- If you are dissatisfied with the company's representative, ask to speak to a supervisor, medical director, or higher authority or the State Insurance Commissioner's Office.
- If you have trouble with a claim, you can contact a Claims Assistance Professional at:

Health Insurance Association of America
202-824-1600
www.hiaa.org

If you need to verify medical and nonmedical personal history, contact the Medical Information Bureau (MIB) and request personal disclosure of medical history. Correct any misinformation.

Medical Information Bureau, Inc.
617-426-3660
www.mib.com

For consumer assistance, contact your State Insurance Department.

Whenever you contact the insurance company, *always* obtain the name of the person you are speaking with, his/her direct telephone extention, date, and the information provided.

*Document everything as you work with
the insurance company.*

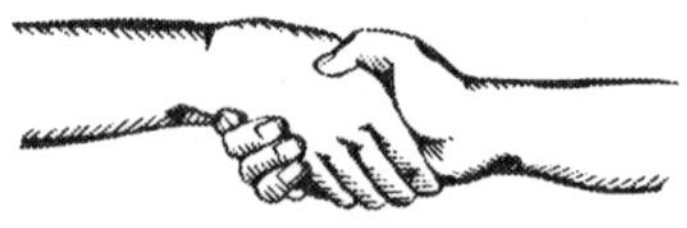

There is a time for everything,
To everything there is a season,
A time to every purpose under the heaven;
A time to be born, and a time to die;
A time to break down, and a time to build up;
A time to keep silent, and a time to speak;
A time to love, and a time to hate;
A time to weep, and a time to laugh;
A time to mourn, and a time to dance;
A time to keep, and a time to cast away.

—Qoheleth (Ecclesiastes) 3:1-3:8

Personal Thoughts

Medicare

What is Medicare?

Medicare is a federal health insurance program that partially pays health costs for people 65 years and older. Certain disabled people under 65 are eligible. Medicare is controlled by the Health Care Financing Administration of the U.S. Department of Health and Human Services. Applications for Medicare are filed at a Social Security Administration office.

How Do You Enroll?

The enrollment process begins three months prior to turning 65 and lasts for a seven-month period. If enrollment is not done at this time, you need to wait for the next open enrollment period. There will be a penalty charge and an increase in premium.

There Are Two Parts to Medicare

Part A—Hospital Portion

Most people do not have to pay a premium for Part A if they have worked enough years prior to receiving this benefit.

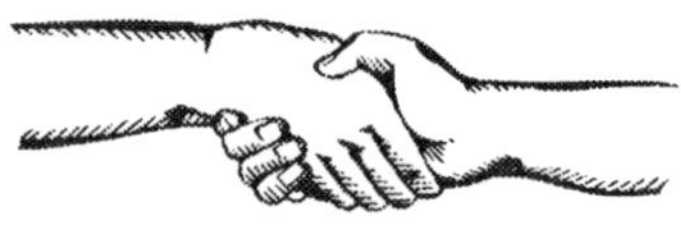

Befriend the people in the billing departments of the physician's office and the insurance company. Ask them to work with you. Marty's medical bills have continued to escalate over six figures. Had he not had Medicare Part A-Part B and Medigap, we would be in extreme financial difficulty. Incidentals alone have cost us a sizeable amount.

— Roz

Personal Thoughts

Benefits:

- Hospital—usually an inpatient deductible. Inquire if the hospital covers this cost.
- Skilled nursing facility.
- Home health care (doctor's prescription) includes nursing and health aide care, therapies, medical supplies, and equipment.
- Hospice care includes nursing, doctor, home aide, services, drugs, therapies, and social services.

Hospital coverage is 90 days each benefit period. A new benefit period begins each time the patient is out of the hospital for 60 days. There is an extra 60 lifetime reserve days.

Part B—Medical Expense Portion

There is a premium, an annual $100 deductible, and 80% coverage of various medical expenses. Many times the preapproved amount is sufficient to cover services.

Benefits:
- Blood
- Clinical laboratory services
- Home health care
- Medical expenses—doctor, surgical supplies, and services
- Medical equipment and supplies
- Outpatient treatment

Prescription and non-prescription drugs are rarely included. Check your area; coverage varies from state to state.

Personal Thoughts

Any Medicare claim that is denied can be disputed. Check the back of the billing information and follow through on any of your disputed claims. Ask your doctor's billing office to help you.

If you turn over your Medicare coverage to an HMO, you may not be eligible for regular Medicare coverage with specific physicians/hospitals in the network.

Yes, This is Important!

- If you are not advised that the service or item is not covered by insurance, you are not responsible for payment. This is known as a waiver of liability notice.
- Medicare statements are mailed once every four weeks. Thoroughly review each statement.
- Do not accept anything that you are not sure is reimbursable. *Check it out first.*
- All procedures and facilities *must* be certified and accepted by Medicare, otherwise, you will be responsible for all bills.
- Medicare does not pay for consumable items, so take the items you have already paid for from the hospital.
- Medicare does not pay for most annual exams or screenings. Check before you go to the doctor.
- VA benefits are not reimbursed by Medicare, but they are reimbursed by Medigap.
- Continuously check for Medicare updates. Contact your nearest Social Security office at: 800-772-1213 (www.ssa.gov) or 800-633-4227 (www.medicare.gov).

Not all doctors accept Medicare payments—
check with your doctor and have them refer only
Medicare-accepting physicians.

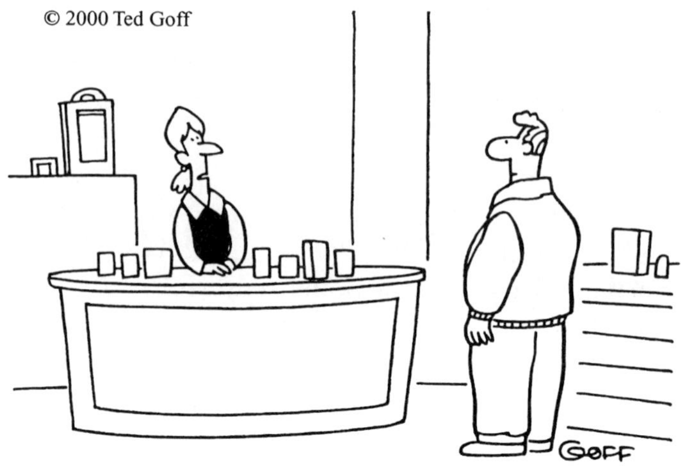

"Sorry, I don't have authorization
to give you good service."

Personal Thoughts

Don't Leave a Gap

Medigap

This is a Medicare supplement sold by some private insurance companies. Medigap becomes the secondary insurance and pays for many expenses not paid by Medicare, but you must have Part B. The first six months that you turn 65 and have Part B of Medicare, there is an open enrollment for Medigap. *This is the only time they cannot refuse you* for any pre-existing condition.

It is very important to contact an insurance agent regarding Medigap. Regulations change constantly.

Information is available by ordering or calling:

Consumer Information Center
800-688-9889
www.pueblo.gsa.gov

Medicare Supplement Insurance
Health Insurance Association of America
202-824-1600
www.hiaa.org

Social Security Administration
800-772-1213
www.ssa.gov

Ask operator to arrange an appointment with your local SSA office.

It is important to pursue and purchase a Medigap policy that fits your needs.

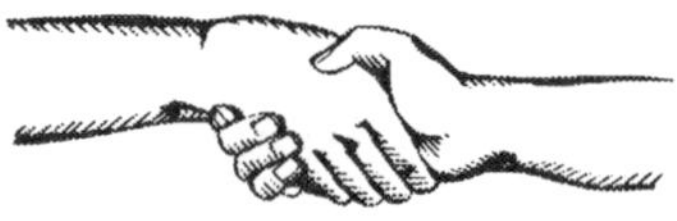

Thank goodness Marty helped save his country. Now they saved us. Marty has monthly appointments with doctors at the VA hospital, as well as his primary physicians at Cedars-Sinai Medical Center. In addition to being in a research program at the VA, he receives most of his medication from their pharmacy. Each prescription is $2, which is a tremendous savings. Check this out! See if you or your spouse are entitled to benefits.

— Roz

Personal Thoughts

____
____
____
____
____
____
____
____
____
____
____
____
____

Department of Veterans Affairs

Don't forget the services the VA offers; they can help.

VA facilities have been updated and many of the physicians divide their time between a notable hospital and the VA facility.

Who Is Eligible?

You and your spouse may be eligible for medical and other benefits or pensions if:

- Service was in any part or division of the military.
- One is a commissioned officer of the Public Health Service.
- One is a commissioned officer of the Environmental Services Administration.
- One is a commissioned officer of the National Oceanic and Atmospheric Administration.
- Service was in a qualifying organization during special periods including World War I and World War II.
- One was in a group that provided military-related services.

How Do We Proceed?

- Call 800-827-1000 to be automatically connected to a VA regional office.
- Bring the following documents: DD214 form, birth certificate, marriage certificate.

Personal Thoughts

- Replacement copies of discharge and separation papers can be obtained by filling out Form 180.
- Counselors are available to help you.
- Receive a copy of *Federal Benefits for Veterans and Dependents* (published yearly).
- If your illness is related to your military service, other benefits may apply.
- Get into the system by seeing a doctor at the VA hospital. Many times your own physician can recommend someone.
- To receive ongoing benefits, the staff will need to become part of your medical treatment team. They will see you on a regular basis and follow your progress with your primary physician.

What Are the Benefits?

Depending on service connection:
- Counseling
- Free/minimal cost of hospitalization
- Free/minimal cost of medical care
- Monetary aid toward burial and headstone costs
- Nursing home care
- Outpatient pharmacy service
- Prosthetic services

Ask for *Federal Benefits for Veterans and Dependents* booklet.

A regional office and medical center are located in central areas throughout each state.

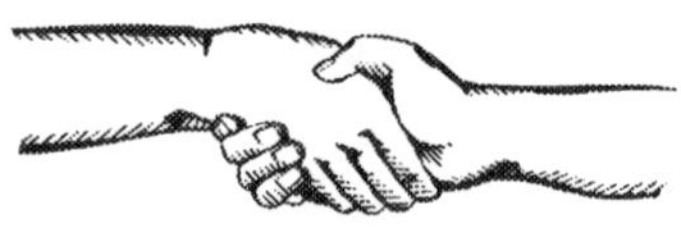

Being able to stay at home with Monty was important to me. Knowing that I was receiving my paycheck and that my job was secure because of the FMLA gave me the security of providing Monty with positive full-time care. If you are eligible for this federal law consider exercising your right. You can take time off from work and your job will be protected.

— Karen

Personal Thoughts

Family Medical Leave Act
(FMLA)

*As a caregiver, you need to be aware of the FMLA.
There may be a time when you will need to change
your work schedule to provide
care to the cancer patient.*

What is FMLA's Purpose?

The purpose of the FMLA is to protect an employee's job and health benefits while taking a leave of absence for health or family needs.

Who Qualifies?

- Employees who work for an eligible FMLA employer.

- Employees who have worked for at least one year; attained 1,250 hours during the previous 12 months; and work for a company with at least 50 employees within a 75-mile radius of the worksite.

- Eligible employers must provide up to 12 weeks of unpaid, job-protected leave and continued health care coverage, to eligible employees.

- The work leave can be intermittent. It does not have to be taken at one time.

- Many employers allow use of sick days and vacation time before utilizing unpaid leave.

- Check with the Human Resources Department of your company regarding the use of sick days and vacation hours.

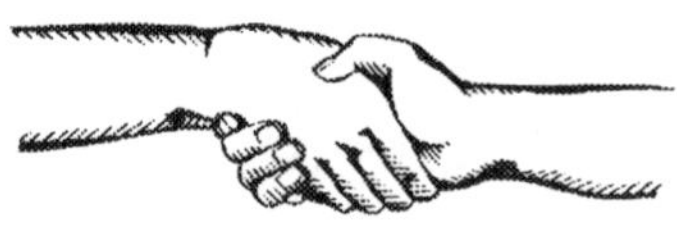

Taking care of Monty while maintaining my regular job duties was extremely difficult. My concentration was with Monty, and I had difficulty focusing on work. The Family Medical Leave Act (FMLA) provided me with an opportunity to stay with Monty. I was able to completely devote my time to him and attend to his needs during the later stage of his illness. Fortunately, my company provided me with a computer so I could telecommute. When Monty was not in need of my immediate attention, I was able to put my efforts toward work.

— Karen

Personal Thoughts

____

____

____

____

____

____

____

____

____

____

Reason for Taking Leave

In the caregiver's case, the Act applies if you are taking care of a spouse, son, daughter, or parent who has a serious health condition such as cancer.

What Are the Job Benefits and Protection?

- The employer must maintain the employee's health coverage under any group health plan during FMLA leave.
- The employee must continue to pay the employee portion of insurance, whenever such insurance was provided before the leave was taken.
- Upon returning from FMLA leave, employees must be restored to their original or equivalent position.
- Equivalent pay, benefits, and other employment terms remain the same.
- The use of the FMLA leave cannot result in the loss of any employment benefit that accrued prior to the start of the employee's leave.

For further information:

U.S. Department of Labor
Wage and Hour Division
800-959-FMLA (800-959-3652)
Provides information on FMLA

The FMLA was created to give flexibility to a caregiver.
Take advantage of this option.

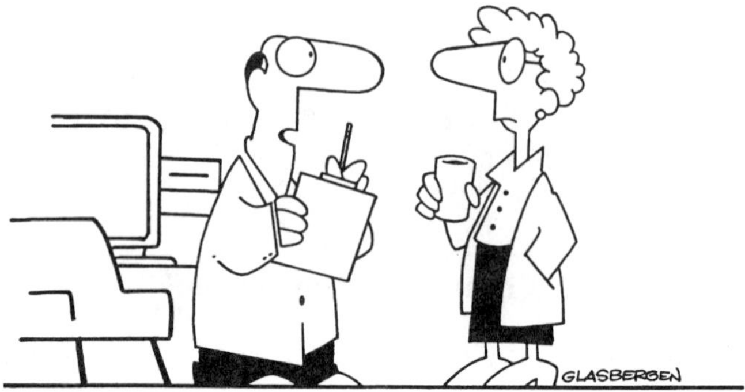

"According to the latest research, the average human body is 20% water and 80% stress."

Personal Thoughts

Fight for Rights

Don't assume that the medical bills you receive are correct.
Check the bills, call the representatives, and write the company.

What Do You Do?

- Remember your rights.
- Be persistent if you have a dispute.
- Write letters.
- Ask your doctor to write letters.
- Ask the benefits department of the patient's company to help.
- Prepare files and keep a copy of *EVERYTHING*.

Other Bills

- Call companies and ask the billing department if you can make arrangements to pay smaller amounts.
- As long as you pay something on a monthly basis, creditors usually do not come after you.
- Retain all of your paperwork.
- People who are persistent and complain usually get positive results.
- Contact a patient advocate agency, if necessary.

Keep detailed records and receipts of claims and expenses.
Consider placing this information on a computer spreadsheet.

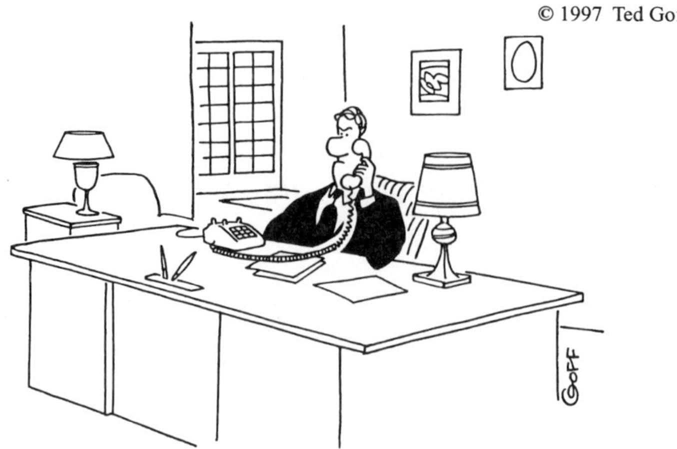

"If you're angry with us, press 1. If you're really angry with us, press 2. If you're really, really angry with us, press 3."

Personal Thoughts

Where Do We File a Complaint?

Insurer	Regulated by
Private Company	State Department of Insurance (found in the Yellow Pages under State Government)
Federally Qualified Health Maintenance (HMO/Kaiser)	U.S. Department of Health/Human Services Division of Compliance
Licensed health care plan service (HMO/Kaiser)	State Department of Corporations, Health Care Service Plan Division
Private employer or union self-insurance	U.S. Department of Labor, Office of Pension/Welfare Benefits
Medicaid	State Department of Social Services
Medicare	U.S. Social Security Administration
Veterans Benefits	Department of Veterans Affairs

HMO comparisons; insurance companies accreditation status	National Committee for Quality and Assurance (NCQA) 800-839-6487
Advocate between and physician	American Association of Patient Health Plans 202-778-3200
Managed care problems	Center for Patient Advocacy 800-846-7444

4

Surviving
The Necessities

Be Proactive

Become familiar on how to research information and learn about the patient's specific cancer!

Available Methods

- Biomedical libraries at universities
- Books
- Clinical trials and cancer research—the NCI continuously sponsors clinical trials:

National Cancer Institute (NCI)

800-4-CANCER (800-422-6237)

www.nci.nih.gov

- Cancer centers
- Oncologist—ask the doctors
- Ask friends for referrals
- Hospital libraries
- Internet
- Literature and booklets from various organizations— usually available in the doctor's office or hospital.
- Magazines, especially health magazines
- Newspapers
- News and talk shows on TV and radio

Monty always brought his updated research to Dr. Shaum. She was very receptive to his findings and willing to investigate and pursue all new treatments and clinical trials. She always went that extra mile to plan Monty's next course of action.

Roz always discussed the latest findings in blood research with Dr. Pepkowitz at the blood facility at Cedars-Sinai Medical Center. It was extremely important to build up Marty's immune system following his stem-cell transplant.

— Roz and Karen

Personal Thoughts

____
____
____
____
____
____
____
____
____
____
____
____

- Specific cancer organizations; see Cancer Resource Guide pages 207-214. Each type of cancer usually has its own organization. The organization will send you free information.

To locate specific organizations call:

CIS part of the NCI
Cancer Information Service
800-4-Cancer (800-422-6237)
www.nci.nih.gov

ACS
American Cancer Society
800-ACS-2345 (800-227-2345)
www.cancer.org

- Support groups: contact a school, hospital, religious organization, or local chamber of commerce.
- Support and donate to cancer organizations. You will be placed on their mailing list and receive the latest cancer research information.
- Talk to other people with the same type of cancer. Ask friends, family, doctor, and American Cancer Society (ACS) for referrals.

The more knowledge, the less fear you will have.

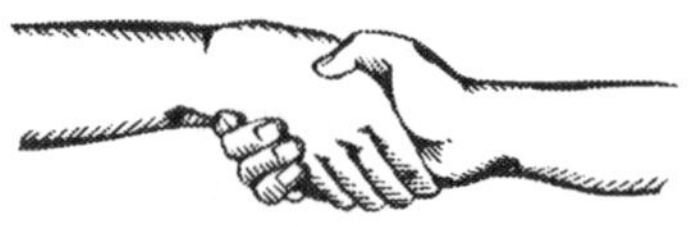

My immediate family members were extremely supportive, especially my brother Jeff and my sister-in-law, Christi. We could always count on their love and support. They made frequent "check in" calls and short visits. I knew if I needed to lean on someone, they would be there for me day or night. Monty's son, brother and his wife were also very supportive. When Monty could not be left alone, I was able to call them and they would be there for Monty. Their constant reliability was extremely supportive for us.

— Karen

Personal Thoughts

Friends and Family

Friends are people you want to hear from.
Family are people who want to hear from you.

How Can Your Friends Help?

Undoubtedly, friends and family will offer you help. If help
is not immediately needed, tell them you appreciate their offer
and will let them know when you do need assistance.
Make a list of the patient's favorite foods and give copies to
friends and family.

- Bring a basket full of "goodies."
- Bring bright floral arrangements.
- Bring books and magazines.
- Bring books on tape.
- Bring lunch to the patient and stay for lunch!
- Bring dinner.
- Bring snacks that are high in calories.
- Bring paper plates and accompaniments.
- Bring relaxation audio tapes.
- Buy subscriptions to a magazine or newspaper.
- Cookie and ice cream deliveries.
- Deliver videos—come back to pick them up.
- Drive the patient to and from medical appointments.

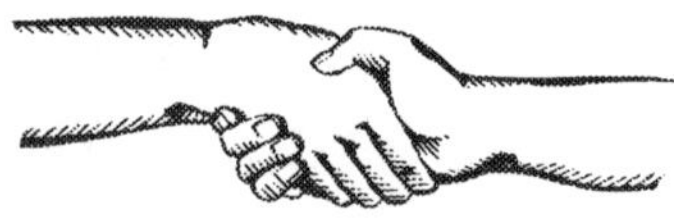

Both Monty and Marty looked forward to daily visits from friends and family. Monty enjoyed deliveries of chocolate chip cookies, sports magazines, and watching baseball games on TV with his friends.

Marty enjoyed reading magazines and watching golf tournaments on TV with his son and friends. He delighted in watching his grandchildren draw pictures while visiting him. We hung pictures around the room along with all his cards.

— Karen and Roz

Personal Thoughts

- Go grocery shopping.
- Help to car pool or drive children to their activities, if necessary.
- If the patient or caregiver has children, offer to babysit.
- Leave a message on the phone or e-mail that you are thinking of them and there is no need to return the phone call.
- Run errands.
- Send dinner from a local restaurant.
- Send humorous and "thinking of you" cards.
- Walk the dog/cat; help care for pets.
- Water the plants.

Honestly sharing your feelings with others can help everyone become more comfortable. Share your feelings of anger, depression, apprehension, and fear. As a caregiver, your friends and family are your support system.

A study at Ohio State University found that the immune system of caregivers was stronger if they were supported with optimistic, warm, generous, nonjudgmental friends and family.

REMEMBER

Positive Energy Creates More Positive Energy.

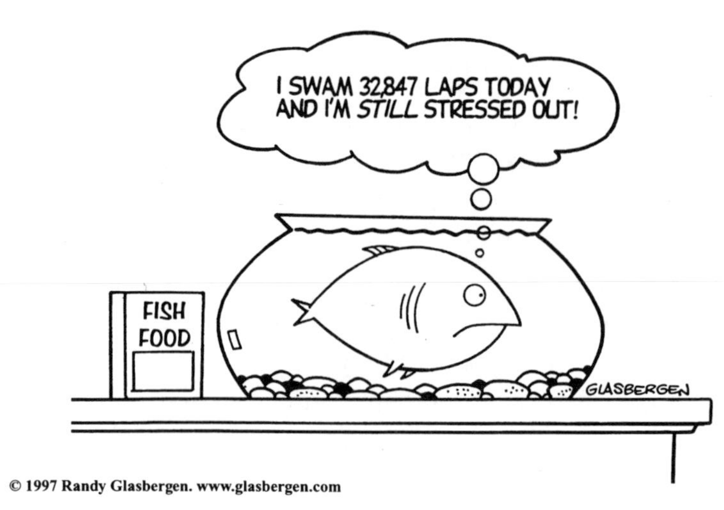

Personal Thoughts

Oh I Would, I Should
Only If I Could
Get Organized

Getting organized will make life a little easier.
Things will become chaotic, so why add more stress
than needed?

What Do You Need to Do?

- Use an organizer or this book.
- Always keep pertinent information on hand, such as:

1. Name of doctors, their specialty, and order of
   relevance.

   ____

   ____

2. Name of contact nurse at each doctor's office.

   ____

   ____

3. Address of doctors.

   ____

   ____

Personal Thoughts

4. Phone, emergency, and fax numbers for all doctors.

____

____

5. Name of insurance billing person at doctor's office.

____

____

6. Hospital phone number.

____

7. Patient's insurance and Social Security numbers.

____

____

8. Pharmacy phone number.

____

9. Home health care number.

____

10. Ambulance number.

____

11. Insurance agent/company phone number and contact
person.

____

____

12. Attorney's name and phone number.

____

____

*Having this information listed on one page will prove
extremely convenient.*

- Keep copies of patient's insurance cards and place them
  in a credit card holder. Keep copies in your wallet.
- Record all doctor appointments, tests, hospital visits,
  treatments, etc.
- Record information pertaining to the patient in between
  doctors' visits. List concerns, questions, appetite, patient's
  symptoms, reaction to medication, new research, etc.
- Keep track of patient's information such as weight, blood
  counts (keep copies), medicine, test results, allergies,
  medical history, etc.

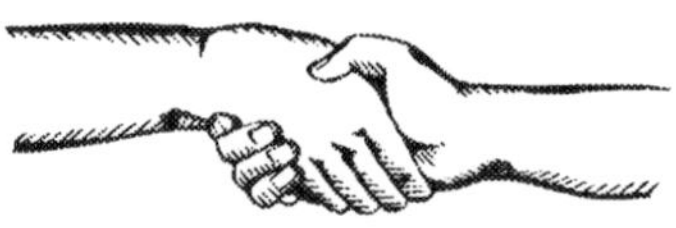

We each purchased a personal organizer. We found this to be the best way to stay organized. Remembering details and appointments became less overwhelming. We used the organizers in addition to our personal writing journals. The organizer consisted of a calendar, priority task list, appointment schedule, address book, extra paper, and a pen. We always tried to take five or ten minutes at the end of the day to write the next day's "to do" list.

— Karen and Roz

Personal Thoughts

- Write or tape-record information during doctor meetings; review it later and take notes in your notebook.

This notebook will be a valuable reference resource.

- Keep all medical records and bills in one area of your home. Use baskets or boxes to hold all information.
- Review and check medical bills as they arrive.
- If there is a question, immediately contact medical provider.
- Organize and keep track of all medical bills. Categorize them by hospital, specific doctor, laboratory, etc.
- Consider utilizing a computer spreadsheet for billing information.
- Encourage the patient to help record information and be proactive.

Remember, the patient may have a monetary cap on his/her insurance for each specific illness, so every amount counts from the beginning.

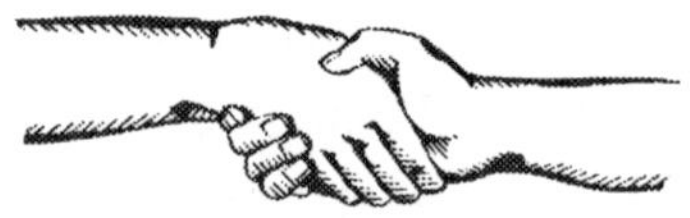

Once we began our journey, I put together the beginnings of what was to become my home away from home...my sack of essentials. I carried this with me at *all* times! As time went along, my bag got heavier and heavier. Initially, my bag consisted of: address book, roll of quarters for phone calls (if I didn't have my cell phone), copies of insurance/medical information, a notepad to write facts or record information from doctors or nurses (at home I would enter this information into my journal).

Many times Monty and I sat in the waiting room for a doctor's appointment or treatment. I was fearful of leaving in case I was needed, so I always packed drinks and snacks. One time while I was at work, Monty had an emergency situation. He called me, and I rushed home and took him to the hospital. Fortunately, I was prepared and had everything I needed, including a change of clothes, in my car.

As a caregiver, being prepared and staying organized helped make my role a little less stressful, and I felt more in control of my situation.

— Karen

A Sack of Essentials

During doctor or hospital visits, your sack of essentials will become a valuable companion.

Essential Items to Pack

- A personal address/phone book.
- A calendar/organizer to write future appointments.
- Copies of important information:
  medical history, medical, social security, and insurance cards . . . *keep these in a credit card holder.*
- A notepad to write important information down and *include questions to ask doctors.*
- A small tape-recorder and blank tapes to record meetings with doctors. Many times you may miss or misunderstand something.
- Things to do requiring...
  minimal concentration:
  magazines, books, puzzles, crafts, small games/cards, radio with headphones, music, books, and self-help tapes.
  maximum concentration:
  mail, bills, necessary to do's.
- Quarters for pay phone, cell phone, or beeper.
  Credit card calls from pay phones are expensive.
- Snacks (use small baggies), drink (freeze a bottle of water and it will stay cold all day).
- Items to refresh yourself with such as wipettes, tissues, brush/comb, make-up, lotion, etc.

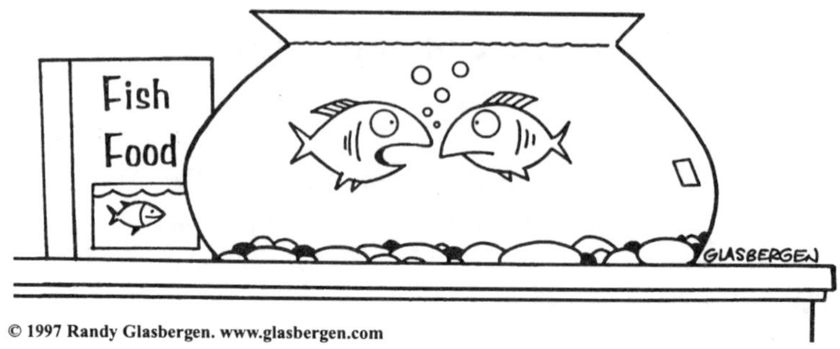

© 1997 Randy Glasbergen. www.glasbergen.com

"If swimming is good for developing shoulders, arms and legs why haven't we developed any shoulders, arms and legs?"

Personal Thoughts

Care for the Caregiver

Do not neglect your own health. If you are concerned about your own physical well-being, consult a physician immediately. You can only effectively take care of someone else if you care for yourself too!

What Can You Do?

- Allow others to help you.
- Day of beauty—manicure/pedicure, new hairdo, facial.
- Daydream..it helps focus and solve problems.
- Do crafts/draw pictures.
- Do jigsaw puzzles.
- Draw a picture/take art classes.
- Eat healthy.
- Exercise/meditation/yoga.
- Go away for a day or the weekend.
- Go to the theater.
- Have a massage.
- Listen to relaxation/music tapes.
- Read a humorous book.
- Read inspirational books.
- Rent movies.
- Spend the evening with a close friend.
- Take a bubble bath.
- Take daily vitamins.
- Visit museums or zoo.

After Marty's sixth operation I felt guilty having so many people waiting around. The waiting room had become an extension of my home, and I felt I had to entertain everyone who was waiting with me. Fortunately my friends are understanding, otherwise I guess they wouldn't be my friends. They allowed me to voice my wants and needs including my desire for company or not. My feelings were always validated by them. This was such an important factor in having a positive support system. Pam and Sheri, my daughters, were always with me, nurturing me, for every one of Marty's 28 surgeries.

— Roz

Personal Thoughts

What Else!

- Accept help from friends and family; allow them to be your support system.
- Ask a friend or relative to fill in for you while you take a break.
- Continue with your outside social engagements.
- Deal with your emotions without feeling guilty...seek professional help if necessary.
- Don't make immediate decisions. Take time and think.
- Don't be afraid to express your feelings.
- Hire someone who can help with household chores, run errands, and stay with the patient.
- Keep a journal—write down your feelings or write letters (not necessarily to send) to relieve tension you are having with anyone.
- Try not to change your daily routine too much; keep your job if you have one (refer to the FMLA page).
- Get dressed everyday. You will feel better.
- Places to find a home helper:
  - Cancer organizations
  - Hospice
  - Oncology office
  - Word of mouth
  - Social worker
  - University nursing school
  - Visiting Nurses Association

Even an hour a day...will sustain your day.
Take time off from CAREGIVING
and
GIVE TO YOURSELF!!

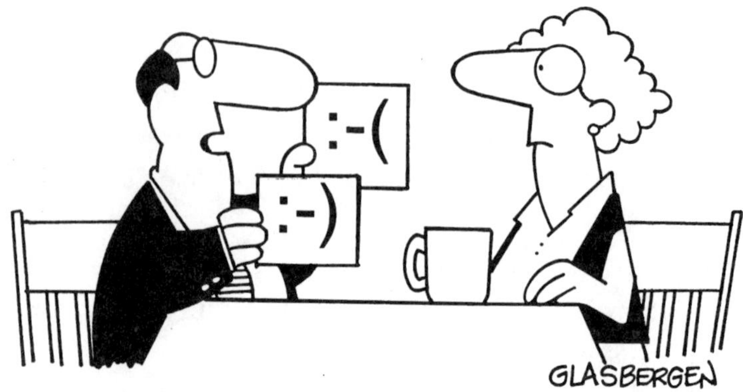

© 1997 Randy Glasbergen. www.glasbergen.com

"You always complain that I don't know how
to show my emotions, so I made these signs."

Personal Thoughts

What Do You Feel?

*You will be swept through an entire range of feelings.
Know that it is normal, try to acknowledge and accept it.*

What Are You Feeling Emotionally?

affectionate	helpful	melancholy
agony	helpless	negative
anticipation	hollow	nervous
anguish	hopeful	numbness
burdened	hostility	puzzled
capable	isolated	separation
disbelieving	lack of interest	shock
disorganized	loneliness	solemn
fear	loss	sympathetic
frustration	loss of control	vulnerable
frustrated	loving	weepy

What Are You Feeling Physically?

achiness	depression	knots in stomach
anxious	detachment	loss/gain weight
backaches	difficulty breathing	low energy
blurred vision	dizziness	panic attacks
can't get out of bed	headaches	sleeplessness
chills	impaired judgment	tension/weakness
colds	knees weak	tightness in throat/chest

Consult your physician if negative symptoms persist.

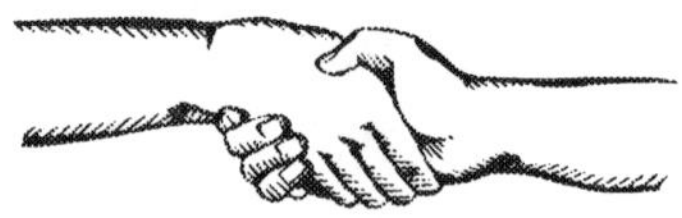

Our situation was unusual because many times our husbands were encountering the same incidents as were we. We had each other to bounce things off. Many nights we would talk on the phone confiding and consoling each other and commiserating about incidents or problems we experienced. It always amazed us how people we did not expect to do something did. On the other hand, some negative occurrences included people who were afraid to visit the hospital for fear of getting sick; wanted to remember the patient as they were before; did not like hospitals; or did what they wanted without considering the patient or the primary caregiver. We realized that many people must face the same things.

We both concluded how difficult it must be for caregivers who have to go it alone and only have people who can sympathize and not empathize!

— Karen and Roz

Personal Thoughts

____

____

____

____

____

____

How Can You Help Yourself?

- Accept disappointment with family or friends.
- Avoid altercations.
- Avoid judgmental and gossipy friends or family.
- Avoid people with negative attitudes.
- Be with people with whom you feel free to convey your thoughts and feelings.
- Confront your feelings.
- Continue with your normal routine as much as possible.
- Do what is comfortable and best for your well-being.
- Don't give up work (see Family Medical Leave Act section).
- Exercise.
- Find a spiritual place.
- Meditate.
- Pray.
- Realize relationships with others will change.
- Seek emotional assistance (group support, chaplain, social worker).
- Set positive goals and write them down.
- Take charge.
- Take care of immediate obligations.
- Take notes on thoughts and questions; this eases your mind.
- Try to be insightful.
- Take walks in comforting and natural surroundings.
- Write in a journal.
- Write "to do" lists and check off as you complete items.

Use positive words, think positive thoughts,
THEN positive feelings and **HOPE** *will follow.*

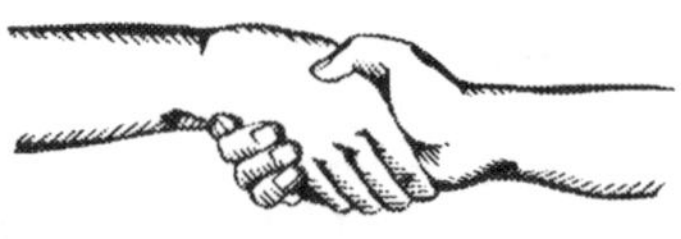

Do not separate yourself from the community.

—*Hillel*

Personal Thoughts

Support Groups

*As much as friends and family try to understand, there is
something special about interacting with people
who are in the same situation, people
who will empathize, not just sympathize.*

What Are the Advantages of a Support Group?

- Allows you to learn more about cancer and treatments.
- Allows you to learn about community resources, organizations, and research.
- Provides you a place to talk and cry without judgment.
- Lets you know that you are not alone.
- Can provide hope as you listen to others explain what they have done and avenues they have pursued.
- Gives hope to you and others.
- Helps you make connections with others who are in the same situation.

Getting the Most Out of the Group

- Align yourself with someone that you can speak to between group sessions.
- Be a good listener—you can benefit from the experiences of others.
- Begin to trust and feel safe within the group so that you can share your feelings and gain benefits of a group setting.
- Don't be judgmental. Be understanding.

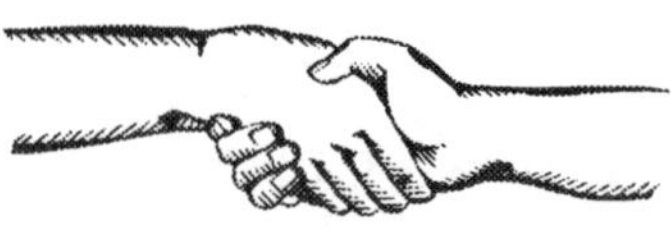

Support groups can be wonderful avenues. Marty and I attended the Wellness Community a few times. While we found it supportive, Marty preferred sharing his feelings with close friends, some of whom had experienced cancer and were quite empathic.

— Roz

Personal Thoughts

- Don't feel obligated to talk.
- Do make an effort to attend every session, even if the cancer patient isn't up to attending his/her group.
- Realize that what you are feeling is often felt by others—even if they haven't stated it.

Other Support People

- Chaplain
- Friends and family
- Internet chat rooms
- Other caregivers
- Psychologist or psychiatrist

How Do You Locate a Support Group?

- Ask at the hospital.
- Ask friends and family.
- Ask the oncologist.
- Ask the social worker in the hospital.
- Call the American Cancer Society to locate an office near you.
- Internet search—refer to resource guide pages 207-214.
- Local newspaper.
- Non-profit social agencies.
- Religious organizations.
- Yellow pages.

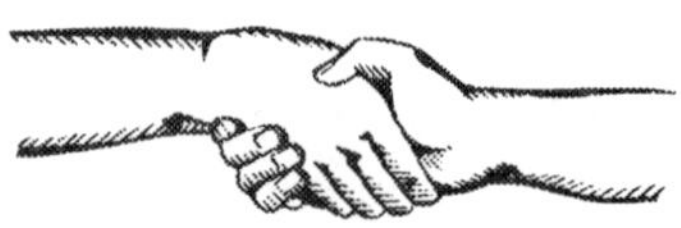

For additional strength and support, Monty and I participated in a support group at the Wellness Community. We found sharing our experiences and exchanging ideas and information to be a very positive weekly experience. Monty had the opportunity to express his emotions, concerns, and feelings with other cancer patients. I was able to share my feelings in the caregivers support group. We developed some wonderful friendships with people in our groups. I am still very good friends with some of the caregivers. We often say, "I love you but wish we had met under different circumstances."

— *Karen*

Personal Thoughts

Organizations

The following organizations can provide information:

National Family Caregivers Association
800-896-3650
www.nfcacares.org

The Wellness Community
888-793-WELL (888-793-9355)
www.wellness-community.org

The Wellness Community provides free psychological support to cancer patients and their families. There are facilities nationwide.

Support groups allow you to share and release your feelings and thoughts safely without condemnation. For the caregiver, as well as the patient, finding other people with the same type of cancer gives you a chance to discuss problems and solutions, find out how others are handling their circumstances, and avail yourself to new resources.

Remember YOU are not alone in caregiving.
Support groups allow others in your situation
to empathize, not just sympathize.

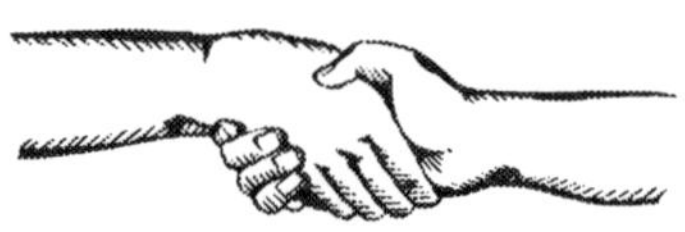

We took advantage of Monty's good days and went on several trips between and during his chemotherapy treatments (he had a constant infusion chemo pack). I always carried my emergency bag and medical records. We were prepared for every emergency that fortunately never happened. We even took two trips to Europe. One of Monty's proudest moments happened during one of these trips. Monty's favorite hobby was making wine in his wine cellar. We were members of a Los Angeles home winemakers group. While in Italy, Monty was notified by our friend Stu that he had won a double gold medal for producing Cabernet Franc from the Adler Winery. This was a momentous occasion and what better place to celebrate then in the wine country of Italy? These are some of my special memories spent with Monty.

— Karen

Personal Thoughts

Vacation Time

Being properly prepared to go away eases any apprehension.

How Do You Prepare?

- Ask your physician for names and phone numbers of qualified doctors in areas you will be visiting.
- Ask for hospitals within the area you are visiting.
- Stay in cities or locations that are near hospitals and doctors.
- Find out how your insurance will apply if there is an emergency.
- Medicare will *not* pay for health care obtained outside the U.S. and its territories; there are limited exceptions for Canada and Mexico.
- Medivac is emergency transportation. Ask your insurance agent or company how this would apply if necessary.
- Bring along a copy of insurance cards and all medical records including latest blood count tests and medical history.
- Bring all medications with you in their original prescription bottles for proper dosage and presciption number.
- Bring along an antibiotic medication.
- Bring prescriptions from your doctor in case of an emergency.
- If using public transportation, do not pack prescriptions in luggage. Keep them with you.

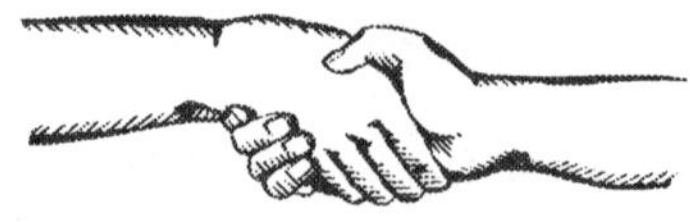

Keeping a Sense of Humor . . . A year after Marty became ill, we decided to take a much-needed vacation. We had just purchased a new sport utility vehicle and were excited to drive it. Our first destination was a national park in Northern California. The day we arrived, however, it was 100 degrees and the roads were being paved. Traffic was at a complete standstill—it took us three long hours to advance 40 miles. Because of the delay, we lost our reservation at a beautiful B&B that we had longed to visit. We ended up staying at a motel. The following evening we went out for dinner, but as we left the restaurant, Marty fell. Not only couldn't he move, he was also bleeding profusely. Luckily I had my emergency bag. I tended to his cuts until the emergency crew arrived. Our choices were to have an ambulance take him to the nearest hospital (a two-hour drive over mountainous roads at night), to helicopter him to Cedars-Sinai, or to carry him back to the hotel room and wait until morning. We opted for the latter. The emergency crew arrived the following morning and carried Marty to our SUV. We drove to Santa Rosa Hospital, where Marty had his hip relocated during an outpatient procedure. Three hours after his operation, we decided to just go home. As we began the five-hour trip, our brand new SUV started puttering. It was Sunday— the day most mechanics have off. We chugged all the way home praying that we wouldn't get stranded on the highway. We were thrilled to arrive home.

— Roz

- Take copies of the following documents: durable power of attorney for health care, power of attorney, and living will, especially if you are going out of the country.
- If traveling overseas, check with patient's doctor regarding traveling conditions and restrictions, water supply, etc.
- Bring your emergency bag with you.

The bag should include:

- adhesive strips
- alcohol wipes
- antacid
- antibiotic ointment

- anti-diarrhea medicine
- change of clothing
- cotton swabs
- disposable gloves
- doctor names, phone numbers
- emergency medications
- hydrogen peroxide
- iodine sticks

- medical insurance cards
- pain relievers
- paper towels
- patient's medical records (copies)

- scissors
- septic stick
- thermometer
- towels
- trash bags
- washcloth
- water bottle
- wipettes

- and any special needs of patient

Assemble small bags of essential items that pertain to your patient. Carry a bag with you each day.

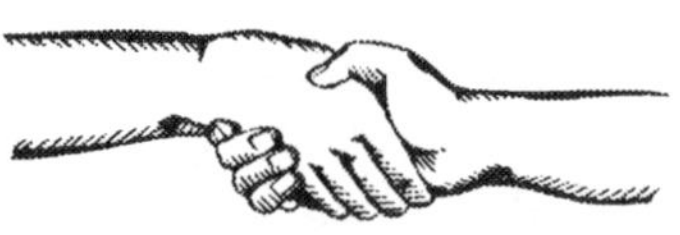

Dear God, I pray for patience. And I want it right now.

— *Oren Arnold*

Personal Thoughts

Do It Now!

Plan a Trip......................Do It Now!

Don't Wait for Later.......Do It Now!

Make a list of all the things that the patient has thought
about doing and............Do It Now!

!!!Do It Now!!!

5

Preparing

For Passage

Be Prepared

Don't depend on physicians to tell you to get personal matters in order. Do this early; you can always make changes later. If the patient becomes incompetent, not able to handle personal affairs, or dies, you will already have everything organized.

Household

- Any leased items (car)
- Deed to house
- Income tax
- Insurance (house, car)
- Mortgage/rent
- Monthly bills
- Property tax
- Utility bills (electricity, telephone, etc.)

Bank Accounts

- Bank Accounts—joint or individual; savings, checking, money market.
- Business Accounts—savings, checking, accounts receivable, etc.
- Location of bank(s).
- Money Market Accounts.
- Identify the authorized signers on each account. If additional signers are needed—*do it now!*

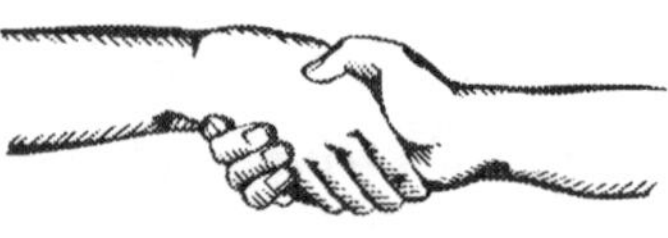

Nothing in life is to be feared. It is only to be understood.

— Marie Curie

Personal Thoughts

General Information

- Military discharge papers, if applicable
- Beneficiary information—make sure it is complete and accurate
- Birth certificate
- Business information
- Credit cards (ask if they will reduce interest payments)
- Deed to burial plot—any pre-arranged instructions
- Divorce Certificate, if applicable
- Durable Power of Attorney for Health Care
- Legal agreements
- Living Will
- Loans
- Marriage Certificate (if applicable)
- Power of Attorney
- Safety deposit boxes
- Social Security records
- Will

Insurance

- Car
- Disability
- Health
- Household
- Life Umbrella policies

Personal Thoughts

Investments

- Bonds
- CDs
- Mutual Funds
- Money Markets
- Stocks

Retirement Funds

- Annuities
- Beneficiaries
- IRA
- Pension

Other

- Miscellaneous Benefits
- Social Security Benefits
- Veteran Benefits

As a caregiver, you must be familiar with these documents. Know where they are located, understand what they are for, make copies and, if necessary, take notes.

It is important that all documents are kept in a safe place and copies are easily available.

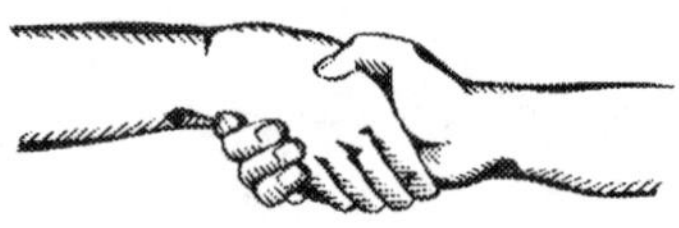

At our hospice agency, a nurse was on call 24 hours a day. Several times, especially in the middle of the night, I needed to call for help. All of the nurses were extremely comforting and were able to handle any situation. Once I called at 1:30 A.M. The nurse informed me that Monty needed a specific pain medication that I did not have. She promptly called the 24-hour hospice pharmacy. The prescription was delivered at 2:45 A.M.

Knowing that someone was there for us at all times was extremely comforting.

— *Karen*

Personal Thoughts

____

____

____

____

____

____

____

____

____

____

Hospice

*Hospice can be a public agency or a private organization
that provides pain relief and supportive services
to the terminally ill patient and the family.
The patient must agree that he/she does not
want to be kept alive on life support.*

When Is It Time for Hospice?

- If the prognosis of life expectancy is six months or less.
- If the patient needs support and symptom control.
- There is no longer a pursuit for a cure or remission.
- The treatment goal is support and comfort.
- The family's need for comfort and support.
- Resuscitation procedures are not administered in Hospice.
- If you call 911 during this period they will be obligated to use life support procedures.

What's the Role of the Hospice Professional?

- Assist in pain management.
- Assist with symptom control for the patient.
- Assist the patient and family with planning a comfortable environment for the patient—be it in the home, hospital, or long-term facility.
- Assess the need of medical supplies for the home, if necessary.
- Bereavement follow-up for survivors.
- Patient and family support—assist in decision making.

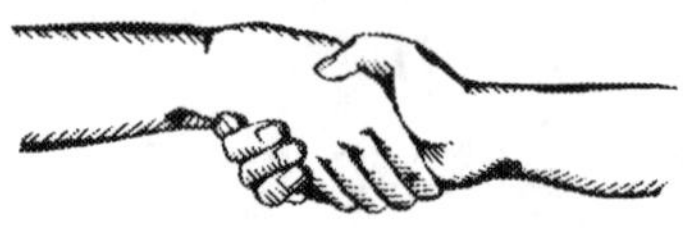

Being able to keep Monty at home during his final weeks was very important to me. I could not have done it without the support of hospice. They provided me with everything I needed to make Monty comfortable. This included medical supplies, prescription drug delivery, a visiting nurse, a social worker, and an attendant.

Their compassion and support were extremely helpful to cope, prepare, and understand the dying process.

— Karen

Personal Thoughts

What Services are Included?

- Chaplains
- Doctors
- Home health aides who care for the patient and do light housework
- Nurses
- Pharmaceutical needs
- Social workers
- Volunteers

For more information contact:

Hospice Education Institute
Hospice Link
800-331-1620
www.hospiceworld.org

National Hospice Organization
800-658-8898
www.nho.org

Children's Hospice International
800-242-4453
www.chionline.org

The oncologist's office and hospital can help set up the Hospice visits for you. *The physician must write the orders for Hospice.*

It is important that the person who visits with you from Hospice is someone you and the patient feel completely comfortable with, so interview people if you can.

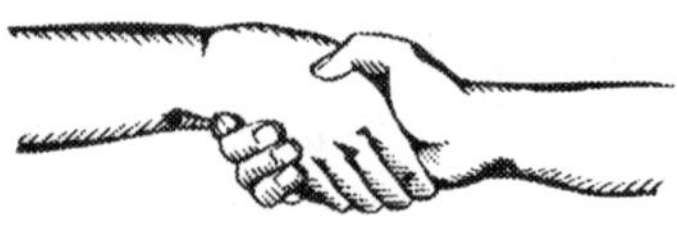

Until death do us part . . . when Dr. Shaum told me that Monty was entering his final days, it was extremely difficult for me to deal with this fact. I had to acknowledge that this was really happening! Fortunately, my dear friend Nancy guided me through this heartwrenching process from her own personal experience. She helped me make the funeral arrangements prior to Monty's death. Although this was a difficult and painful experience, it gave me the opportunity to concentrate on exploring my options in a timely manner and not deal with any last minute decisions. This made coping somewhat easier.

— *Karen*

Personal Thoughts

Final Preparations

This is a topic people do not wish to discuss or consider, but cancer gives one an opportunity to plan ahead.

What Can We Do?

- Be aware of conflicting emotions and feelings, guilt, anger, futility, love, hope, tears, numbness, etc.
- Chaplains and professional counselors can help.
- Discuss religious and spiritual beliefs, customs, and preferences of the service.
- Express and share feelings—communication and honesty are important and can be very consoling.
- Read literature and books pertaining to the process of dying.
- Purchase a cemetery plot.
- Purchase necessary funeral items in advance.
- Some cemeteries have funeral directors to help with arrangements.
- Visit with an estate planning attorney.

It is best for all concerned to make preparations beforehand so rational decisions can be made and turbulence can be avoided.

Bereavement support groups are important. Find a group you are comfortable with by interviewing and observing.

6

Knowledge
Increases Strength

Cancer Resource Guide

Cancer organizations are available to answer questions and supply information. Take advantage of these resources.

General Cancer Information

American Cancer Society (ACS)

National Headquarters
1599 Clifton Road NE
Atlanta, GA 30329
404-320-3333
800-ACS-2345
(800-227-2345)
www.cancer.org

National Cancer Institute (NCI)

9000 Rockville Pike
Bethesda, MD 20892
301-496-5803
800-4-CANCER
(800-422-6237)
www.nci.nih.gov

Cancer Information Service (CIS)

31 Center Drive, MSC2580
Building 31, Room 10A07
Bethesda, MD 20892
800-4-CANCER
(800-422-6237)
www.cis.nci.nih.gov

CancerNet

www.cancernet.nci.nih.gov

CancerFax

301-402-5874
E-mail:
cancermail@icicc.nci.nih.gov

Candlelighters Childhood Cancer Foundation

3910 Warner Street
Kensington, MD 20895
301-962-3520
800-366-2223
www.candlelighters.org

The National Children's Cancer Society

1015 Locust Street, Suite 600
St. Louis, MO 63101-1323
314-241-1600
800-5-FAMILY
(800-532-6459)
www.children-cancer.com

Specific Cancer Organizations

American Brain Tumor Association

2720 River Road, Suite 146
Des Plaines, IL 60018
847-827-9910
800-886-2282
www.abta.org

National Brain Tumor Foundation

414 Thirteenth Street, Suite 700
Oakland, CA 94612
510-839-9777
800-934-CURE
(800-934-2873)
www.braintumor.org

National Alliance of Breast Cancer Organizations (NABCO)

9 East 37th Street, 10th Floor
New York, NY 10016
888-80-NABCO
(888-806-2226)
800-719-9154
www.nabco.org

Susan G. Komen Breast Cancer Foundation

5005 LBJ Freeway, Suite 370
Dallas, TX 75244
972-855-1600
800-I'M AWARE
(800-462-9273)
www.breastcancerinfo.com
www.komen.org

Cathy's Esophageal Cancer Cafe

www.tzet.com/wolfgram/ec/cafe

Y-ME National Breast Cancer Organization

212 W. Van Buren, 4th Floor
Chicago, IL 60607
312-986-8338
800-221-2141 (English)
800-986-9505 (Spanish)
www.y-me.org

Ovarian Cancer National Alliance

910 17th Street NW
Washington, DC 20006
202-331-1332
www.ovariancancer.org

Kidney Cancer Association

1234 Sherman Avenue,
Suite 203
Evanston, IL 60202
847-332-1051
800-850-9132
www.nkca.org

Leukemia & Lymphoma Society

600 Third Avenue
New York, NY 10016
212-573-8484
800-955-4LSA
(800-955- 4572)
www.leukemia-lymphoma.org

American Lung Association

1740 Broadway, 14th Floor
New York, NY 10019-4374
212-315-8700
800-LUNG-USA
(800-586-4872)
www.lungusa.org

**Lymphoma Research
Foundation of America**

8800 Venice Blvd., Suite 207
Los Angeles, CA 90034
310-204-7040
800-500-9976
www.lymphomafocus.org

**The International Myeloma
Foundation**

2129 Stanley Hills Drive
Los Angeles, CA 90046
323-654-3023
800-452-CURE
(800-452-2873)
www.myeloma.org

**Caitlin Raymond
International Registry**

(Coordination center for those in
need of bone marrow or cord
blood transplants)
University of Massachusetts
Medical Center
55 Lake Avenue North
Worcester, MA 01655
508-334-8969
800-726-2824
www.crir.org

**National Bone Marrow
Transplant Link**

20411 West 12 Mile Road,
Suite 108
Southfield, MI 48076
800-LINK-BMT
(800-546-5268)
http://comnet.org/nbmtlink

**Transplant Recipients
International
Organization, Inc. (TRIO)**

1000 Sixteenth Street NW,
Suite 602
Washington, DC 20036
202-293-0980
800-TRIO-386
(800-874-6386)
www.trioweb.org

Cancer Support Groups

**National Coalition for
Cancer Survivorship (NCCS)**

1010 Wayne Ave, Seventh Floor
Silver Springs, MD 20910
877-NCCS-YES
(877-622-7937)
www.cansearch.org

Wellness Community

National Headquarters
35 East 7th Street, Suite 412
Cincinnati, OH 45205
888-793-WELL
(888-793-9355)
www.wellness-community.org

National West Coast Office

2716 Ocean Park Blvd.,
Suite 1040
Santa Monica, CA 90405
310-314-2555
www.la.wellnesscommunity.org

Cancer Care, Inc.

National Office
275 Seventh Avenue
New York, NY 10001
212-302-2400
800-813-HOPE
(800-813-4673)

Cancer Hope Network

Two North Road, Suite A
Chester, NJ 07930
877-HOPE-NET
(877-467-3638)
www.cancerhopenetwork.org

Gilda's Club

195 West Houston Street
New York, NY 10014
212-647-9700
888-GILDA 4 U
(888-445-3248)
www.gildasclub.org

**Coping With Cancer
Magazine**

P.O. Box 682268
Franklin, TN 37068
615-790-2400
www.copingmag.com

**National Family Caregivers
Association**

10400 Connecticut Ave.,
Suite 500
Kensington, MD 20895
www. nfcacares.org

**Partnership for Caring
Choice in Dying**

(Advanced Directives)
National Office
1035 30th Street NW
Washington, DC 20007
202-338-9790
800-989-WILL
(800-989-9455)
www.choices.org

Compassion in Dying

(Advocates for pain management and end of life options)
6312 SW Capitol Highway,
Suite 415
Portland, OR 97201
503-221-9556
www.compassionindying.org

**Hospice Education Institute
Hospice Link**

190 Westbrook Road
Essex, CT 06426
860-767-1620
(800-331-1620)
www.hospiceworld.org

**National Hospice
Organization (NHO)**
1700 Diagonal Road,
Suite 300
Alexandria, VA 22314
703-243-5900
800-658-8898
www.nho.org

**Ronald McDonald
House Charities**
One McDonald's Drive
Oak Brook, IL 60523
630-623-7048
www.rmhc.com

**Children's Hospice
International**
2202 Mount Vernon Avenue,
Suite 3C
Alexandria, VA 22301
703-684-0226
800-2-4-CHILD
(800-242-4453)
www.chionline.org

**Burger King Cancer
Caring Center**

4117 Liberty Avenue
Pittsburgh, PA 15224
412-622-1210
www.trfn.clpgh.org/cancercaring

**National Association of
Hospital Hospitality
Houses, Inc.**

P.O. Box 18087
Ashville, NC 28814
800-542-9730
www.NAHHH.org

**American Society of
Clinical Oncology (ASCO)**

225 Reinekers Lane,
Suite 650
Alexandria, VA 22314
703-299-0150
www.asco.org

Research Groups

*These groups focus on research.
Visit their website for the latest
information or call them.*

**American Institute for
Cancer Research (AICR)**
1759 R Street NW
202-328-7744
800-843-8114
www.aicr.org

**Israel Cancer Research Fund
(ICRF)**
8383 Wilshire Boulevard,
Suite 341
Beverly Hills, CA 90211
323-651-1200
E-mail: *icrfla@aol.com*

Stop Cancer
1875 Century Park East,
Suite 1740
Los Angeles, CA 90067
310-286-2511
www.stopcanceronline.org

Air Transportation for Cancer Patients

National Patient Travel Center

4620 Haygood Road, Suite 1
Virginia Beach, VA 23455
757-318-9174
800-296-1217
www.PatientTravel.org

AirLifeLine National Office

50 Fullerton Court, Suite 200
Sacramento, CA 95825
916-641-7800
800-446-1231
877-AIRLIFE (877-247-5433)
www.airlifeline.org

Complementary and Alternative Medicine Organizations

National Center for Complementary and Alternative Medicine (NCCAM)

NCCAM Clearinghouse
P.O. Box 8218
Silver Springs, MD 20907
888-644-6226
http://nccam.nih.gov

University of Texas Houston Health Science Center Center for Alternative Medicine

1515 Holcombe Blvd.
Houston, TX 77030
800-392-1611
www.sph.uth.tmc.edu/utcam

Cancer Control Society
(Provides a non-toxic therapy and diagnostic test directory)
2043 N. Berendo St
Los Angeles, CA 90027
323-663-7801

American Association of Oriental Medicine

433 Front Street
Catasauqua, PA 18032
610-266-1433
888-500-7999
www.aaom.org

American Dietetic Association

216 W. Jackson
Chicago, IL 60606
800-366-1655
www.eatright.org

American Herbalists Guild

P.O. Box 70
Roosevelt, UT 84066
435-722-8434
www.healthy.net/herbalists

Other Informative Websites

Oncologist Link

www.oncolink.upenn.edu

Cancer Directory

www.cancerdirectory.com

Healthon/WebMD

www.webmd.com

Medicine Information

www.cancerlinks.org
www.rxlist.com

American Red Cross

800-448-3543
www.redcross.org
Enter your zipcode for a local
agency.

**Pertinent Consumer
Insurance and Medical
Advice Centers**

**Medical Information
Bureau, Inc.**

160 University Avenue
Westwood, MA 02090
617-426-3660
www.mib.com

**Department of Health
and Human Services**

200 Independence Avenue SW
Washington, DC 20201
202-619-0257
877-696-6775
www.os.dhhs.gov

National Library of Medicine

8600 Rockville Pike
Bethesda, MD 20894
800-FIND-NLM
(888-346-3656)
www.nim.nih.gov

**Consumer Information
Center**

Dept. 33
Pueblo, CO 81009
800-638-6833
www.pueblo.gsa.gov

**National Insurance
Consumer Hotline**

1001 Pennsylvania Avenue NW
Washington, DC 20004
800-942-4242

**American Association of
Health Plans**

(Advocate between patients
and physicians)
1129 20th Street NW, Suite 600
Washington, DC 20036
202-778-3200
Fax: 202-331-7487
www.aahp.org

National Committee for Quality Assurance

2000 L Street NW, Suite 500
Washington, DC 20036
202-955-3500
800-839-6487
www.ncqa.org

Center for Patient Advocacy

1350 Beverly Road, Suite 108
McLean, VA 22101
703-748-0400
800-846-7444
www.patientadvocacy.org

Family Medical Leave Act (FMLA)

U.S. Department of Labor
Wage & Hour Division
200 Constitution Avenue NW
Washington, DC 20210
800-959-FMLA
(800-959-3652)

Social Security Administration

U.S. Department of Health and
Human Services Social Security
800-772-1213
www.ssa.gov

American Association of Retired Persons (AARP)

601 E Street NW
Washington, DC 20049
800-424-3410
www.aarp.org

Medicare/Medigap

800-Medicare (800-633-4227)
www.medicare.gov

U.S. Department of Veteran Affairs

800-827-1000
www.va.gov

Disabled American Veterans

807 Maine Avenue SW
Washington, DC 20024
202-554-3501
www.dav.org

Health Insurance Association of America

555 13th Street NW
Washington, DC 20004
202-824-1600
www.hiaa.org
VA regional office
800-827-1000

U.S. Senate Special Committee on Aging

202-224-5364
www.senate.gov/~aging

This list of resources is provided for your convenience. It is to be used for reference only. Personally contact an organization, research group, or comprehensive center for specific information. All data was updated at time of printing.

National Cancer Institute (NCI) Designated Comprehensive Cancer Centers

The following are National Cancer Institute (NCI) designated Comprehensive Cancer Centers. These centers are recognized by the NCI after meeting certain criteria designated by a National Comprehensive Cancer Network (NCCN) core membership group. The NCCN centers develop and set standards of care for the treatment of cancer with the goal of providing high-quality, cost-effective services to cancer patients. These comprehensive centers conduct early phase, innovative research and clinical trials, and provide outreach educational programs and information on cancer to the community.

Alabama
University of Alabama at Birmingham
Birmingham, AL 35293
205-934-5077

Arizona
Arizona Cancer Center University of Arizona
Tucson, AZ 85724
520-626-7925

California
Beckman Research Institute City of Hope
Duarte, CA 91010
626-301-8164

Jonsson Comprehensive Cancer Center University of California Los Angeles
Los Angeles, CA 90095
310-825-5268

USC/Norris Comprehensive Cancer Center University of Southern California
Los Angeles, CA 90033
323-865-0876

Chao Family Comprehensive Cancer Center University of California at Irvine
Orange, CA 92868
714-456-6310

**UCSF Cancer Center
& Cancer
Research Institute**
University of California San
Francisco
San Francisco, CA 94115
415-502-1710

Colorado
**University of Colorado Cancer
Center**
Denver, CO 80262
303-315-3007

Connecticut
**Yale University School of
Medicine**
New Haven, CT 06520
203-785-4371

**District of Columbia
Lombardi Cancer Research
Center
Georgetown University
Medical Center**
Washington, DC 20007
202-687-2110

Illinois
**University of Chicago Cancer
Research Center**
Chicago, IL 60637
773-702-6180

**Robert H. Lurie Cancer
Center
Northwestern University**
Chicago, IL 60611
312-908-5250

Maryland
**John Hopkins Oncology
Center**
Baltimore, MD 21287
410-955-8822

Massachusetts
Dana-Farber Cancer Institute
Boston, MA 02115
617-632-2155

Michigan
University of Michigan
Ann Arbor, MI 48109
734-936-1831

**Barbara Ann Karmanos
Cancer Institute
Wayne State University**
Detroit, MI 48201
313-993-7777

Minnesota
**University of Minnesota
Cancer Center**
Minneapolis, MN 55455
612-624-8484

Mayo Clinic Cancer Center
Rochester, MN 55905
507-284-3753

New Hampshire
**Norris Cotton Cancer Center
Dartmouth-Hitchcock Medical
Center**
Lebanon, NH 03756
603-650-6300

New York
Albert Einstein College of Medicine
Bronx, NY 10461
718-430-2302

Roswell Park Cancer Institute
Buffalo NY 14263
716-845-2389

Kaplan Cancer Center
New York University Medical Center
New York, NY 10016
212-263-6485

Memorial Sloan-Kettering Cancer Center
New York, NY 10021
212-639-6561

Herbert Irving Comprehensive Cancer Center
Columbia University
New York, NY 10032
212-305-8602

North Carolina
University of North Carolina Lineberger Comprehensive Cancer Center
Chapel Hill, NC 27599
919-966-3036

Duke Comprehensive Cancer Center
Durham, NC 27710
919-684-5613

Wake Forest University Bowman Gray School of Medicine
Winston-Salem, NC 27157
336-716-7971

Ohio
Ireland Cancer Center Case Western Reserve University and University Hospitals of Cleveland
Cleveland, OH 44106
216-844-8562

Arthur G. James Cancer Hospital Ohio State University
Columbus, OH 43210
614-293-7518

Pennsylvania
University of Pennsylvania Cancer Center
Philadelphia, PA 19104
215-662-6065

Fox Chase Cancer Center
Philadelphia, PA 19111
215-728-2781

University of Pittsburgh Cancer Institute
Pittsburgh, PA 15213
412-692-4670

Texas
M.D. Anderson Cancer Center
Houston, TX 77030
713-792-6000

San Antonio Cancer Institute
San Antonio, TX 78229
210-616-5580

Vermont
Vermont Cancer Center
University of Vermont
Burlington, VT 05405
802-656-4414

Washington
Fred Hutchinson Cancer
Research Center
Seattle, WA 98104
206-667-4305

Wisconsin
Comprehensive Cancer Center
University of Wisconsin
Madison, WI 53792
608-263-8610

Glossary

Abnormal	That which deviates from the normal.
Adenocarcinoma	A type of cancer involving the cells that line the walls of various body organs.
Adjuvant Therapy	Treatment given in addition to the primary treatment to effectively treat and increase the possibility of remission/cure, such as radiation, chemotherapy, hormonal, or immunotherapy.
Allogeneic	The infusion of bone marrow from one individual (donor) to another.
Alopecia	The loss of hair throughout the body.
Anemia	A decrease in the number of red blood cells producing tiredness, shortness of breath, and weakness.
Antiemetic	A drug that prevents or controls nausea and vomiting.
Antimetabolites	Anticancer drugs that interfere with the process of DNA production to prevent cell division.
Antigen	Any substance that causes the body to produce natural antibodies.
Antineoplastic Agent	A drug that prevents, kills or blocks the growth and spread of cancer cells.
Asymptomatic	No obvious symptoms/signs of the disease although cancer is detected via tests. Cure statistics are very high.

Atypical	Abnormal; in cancer the cell division process is "atypical."
Autologous	The infusion of a patient's own bone marrow which has been previously taken and stored.
Benign Tumor	A growth that is abnormal. It is not cancerous and does not spread.
Bilateral	Both sides of the body are affected.
Biopsy	A small piece of tissue is surgically removed for microscopic examination.
Blood Cells	Microscopic structures made in the bone marrow consisting of red blood cells, white blood cells, and platelets.
Blood Count	Determines the number of white blood cells, red blood cells and platelets in a sample of blood taken from the body.
Bone Marrow	Blood cells are manufactured in this soft, fatty filling of bone cavity.
Brain Scan	Radioactive dye is injected into the vein so brain images can be recorded. This is rarely done today. A CT scan or MRI is the usual procedure.
Cancer	More than 100 types of diseases which are identified by the abnormal growth and spread of abnormal cells. Some cells form tumors and invade surrounding tissue or spread through the bloodstream or the lymph system to other parts of the body.

Carcinoma — A type of cancer that develops in tissues that cover or line organs of the body.

Central Venous Catheter — A special intravenous tubing that is inserted surgically into a large vein near the heart and exiting through another area of the body allowing medications, blood products or fluids to be given and samples to be taken.

Cell — The basic structure of living matter consisting of a cell wall, a nucleus in the center surrounded by cytoplasm.

Chemotherapy — Introducing one or a combination of anticancer drugs through intravenous methods. Side effects may occur. There is medication for nausea.

Clinical Trial — Potentially effective drug treatment for patients but still under scientific investigation. Some insurance companies will not cover clinical trial experiments.

Code Blue — An alarm set off by medical staff when a patient has suffered either cardiac pulmonary or respiratory arrest.

Combined Modality Therapy — Combining and alternating different types of treatment to aggressively attack cancer cells.

Computerized Tomography Scan — Highly transmitted specialized X-ray studies that can find cancer. Usually referred to as CT or CAT scans.

Cyst — An abnormal saclike structure that contains liquid. It may be benign or malignant.

| **Diagnosis** | Identifying the disease by the professional. |

Diagnosis   Identifying the disease by the professional.

DNA   Part of the nucleus of all cells showing genetic information of the cell growth, function, and division.

Endoscopy   A procedure using a tube-like instrument for a biopsy to see certain areas of the body.

Frozen Section   In a biopsy, tissue is removed, frozen, sliced thin, stained and examined under a microscope.

Hematocrit (HCT)   The percentage of red blood cells in the blood.

Hormones   Secretion by certain organs helping to regulate growth, metabolism, and reproduction. Sometimes hormones are given as treatment.

Immunotherapy   Artificial stimulation of the immune system to treat or fight disease.

Infusion   Delivering fluids or medications into the blood stream intravenously over a period of time.

Interferon   A body protein made by normal cells that can fight/stop cancer cell growth. It can also be artificially produced.

Localized Cancer   Cancer which has not spread and is contained at site of origin.

Lymph   The clear fluid that circulates throughout the body containing white blood cells and antibodies.

Lymphocytes	Part of the white blood cell that kills viruses and defends against the invasion of foreign material.
Magnetic Resonance Imaging	A procedure using magnetic fields to show images of the body. Usually referred to as MRI.
Malignant Tumor	A mass of cancer cells that can spread to other parts.
Metastasis	New cancer sites where the cancer cells have spread to other areas of the body through the lymph system or bloodstream.
Mitosis	Cell reproduction process.
Myelosuppression	A decrease in the production of white blood cells, red blood cells, and platelets by the bone marrow.
Neoplasm	A new abnormal growth.
Neutropenia	A decreased number of neutrophils, a type of white blood cell that fights infection.
Nodule	A small mass which can be cystic or solid.
Nuclear Scan	A radioactive substance tracer is injected into the bloodstream and a machine then takes pictures over the area.
Oncologist	A physician who specializes in the diagnosis and treatment of cancer. There are also certified nurses who have specialized in the education and treatment of cancer patients.

Palliative Treatment	Improving the quality of life by relieving symptoms, but doesn't change the course of the disease.
Pathology	Studying the disease through a microscopic examination of the tissues and organs of the body.
Petechiae	Small areas of bleeding under the skin, usually due to a low platelet count.
Platelet	Found in the blood to help clotting. A normal platelet count usually ranges between 140.–440. K/ul.
Prognosis	Predicting the path of the disease and the life expectancy.
Radioactive Implant	High dose radiation that is put into/around the cancer cell to kill it.
Radiotherapy	Treating cancer with high energy radiation to shrink or destroy the cancer cell.
Red Blood Cells (Erythrocyte)	Cells in the blood that bring oxygen to tissues and take carbon dioxide from them.
Regional Cancer	Spread of the cancer to the surrounding area of original site, but confined to only one area of the body.
Relapse	The reappearance of cancer after a disease-free period.
Remission	A period of time when the signs or symptoms of the cancer has disappeared, responding to the treatment. This is not necessarily a cure.

Sarcoma	A malignant tumor of muscles or connective tissues such as bone and cartilage.
Secondary Tumor	A tumor that has developed as a result of the spread of the original cancer cell.
Staging	Evaluating the extent and degree of the disease for treating and determining prognosis.
Stoma	An opening in the body which has been surgically made.
Systemic disease	A disease that affects the whole body instead of a specific organ.
Tissue	Collection of cells that are similar.
Thrombocytopenia	A low number of platelets, which may cause bleeding.
Tumor	An abnormal tissue mass.
Ultrasound	High frequency sound waves used to locate a deep tumor in the body. Known as ultrasonography.
White Blood Cells (WBC)	Cells in the blood that are responsible for fighting germs, infections, and allergy-causing agents. Granulocytes and lymphocytes are part of the white blood cells. A normal white blood cell count usually ranges between 4.1 - 10.0 K/ul.
X-ray	Picture taken through high energy radiation. Low doses are used to diagnosis diseases and high doses to treat cancer.

Personal Thoughts

Share Your Secret
Tip Us Off

Cancer never takes a vacation, which means you, as a caregiver, are always on call. It has been our experience that interacting and sharing with others helps ease your journey.

Do you have a caregiver tip to share?

If you would like to share your tip with other caregivers, write or e-mail us. We may include your tip in a future edition and list your name as a contributor.

Cancer Caregivers

P.O. Box 642777

Los Angeles, CA 90064

www.cancercaregivers.com

e-mail: tips@cancercaregivers.com

The Rainy Day

Be still, sad heart
*   And cease repining;*
Behind the clouds
*   Is the sun still shining;*
Thy fate is the
*   Common fate of all,*
Into each life
*   Some rain must fall,*
Some days must be
*   Dark and dreary.*

—Henry Wadsworth Longfellow

The Authors

Karen Kirzner Adler

Karen Kirzner Adler is originally from New Hampshire. After two years at Boston University she relocated to California where she completed her education at San Diego State University receiving her B.S. in liberal studies. In graduate school, she pursued her California teaching credentials. Karen taught elementary school and children with learning disabilities in Los Angeles.

Karen left the teaching profession to become an event planner. Her job consisted of organizing seminars and training seminar speakers, which often led to her own speaking engagements. Karen moved to the Human Resources Department of a large organization where she trained company employees. Presently she works in Human Resources in the entertainment industry in Los Angeles.

Following a two-year battle with esophageal cancer, Karen's husband Monty died in 1997. Realizing the limited amount of information available to cancer caregivers, Karen felt the necessity to write this book and share her knowledge and experiences. Karen and Monty met in 1978 and married in 1988.

Rozlyn Forman Kleiman

Rozlyn Forman Kleiman's interest has always been in the educational field; she taught early education and special needs students in New York, Ohio, Florida, and California. Her undergraduate work was completed at Adelphi University in New York. She received her M.Ed. degree specializing in learning disabilities from the University of Cincinnati and obtained an M.A. degree in Art Therapy/Marriage, Family, and Child Counseling from Loyola Marymount in Los Angeles. In 1989 Rozlyn became active in the fight against AIDS and was Vice-President and board member for an AIDS organization in Los Angeles. Besides arranging outings and parties for children with AIDS, she conducted family art therapy and counseling sessions. She is on the board of Camp Pacific Heartland, a camp for children with AIDS and their siblings. Rozlyn teaches Sunday School to children with special needs. Presently she is also the proprietor of the Studio Salon located at a major movie studio in Los Angeles.

In addition to Marty, Rozlyn has provided caregiving to other family members who have suffered due to automobile accidents and surgery. All of her caregiving experience inspired Rozlyn to write this book. Her husband Marty was diagnosed with multiple myeloma over five years ago and together they have survived his cancer. Marty and Roz married in 1983 and have five children and seven grandchildren.

"The Gift of Life"

Nowadays, when people ask me what I got for the holidays, I tell them "The Gift of Life." I received something that all the money in the world couldn't buy.

I was the patriarch of my family. I took care of everyone—emotionally and financially. Then at 68 years old, I was diagnosed with terminal cancer— multiple myeloma and had 27 surgeries. I was forced to become dependent upon my physicians, hospital staff, my wife Roz, and my family. I was hospitalized for six months. I had a bone marrow transplant and wound up in ICU four times. One time I actually died for 30 seconds and came back. My family stayed by my side continuously. Their love and support encouraged me to fight.

After being released from the hospital, I was bedridden at home for 12 months . . . the care from Roz and my family intensified. Roz became my closest companion and my nurse. Unable to perform normal daily life tasks or function physically in any way, the unconditional support, assistance and loving care of my wife and family gave me a tremendous amount of courage. I was able to battle and conquer this dreaded disease. My wife had to learn all the necessary caregiving requirements to help nurse me.

My faith in God was extolled by the Rabbi's constant visits at the hospital. I attended services at the hospital every year since I was diagnosed. The first year they wheeled me down on a hospital bed, the second year I used a wheelchair, the third year I walked up to the podium with a cane and told my story, and then finally I walked on my own.

It's been five years since I was told I had cancer. I'm pleased to say that with the support of those around me—my wife, my children and grandchildren and my doctors—I am able to work, play golf, travel, and do most of all the normal tasks I used to do. Obviously I can't run the 10K marathon, but I don't think I could have before the cancer either! I have been blessed with a second chance at life and I cherish that.

Unfortunately Monty did not have this chance but I do know, because we spoke about this often, if it were not for our wives and their unconditional love, support, and caring neither one of us would have had the quality of care that we received. I was always amazed how Monty packed his IVs and went off trekking through Europe; this could not have been done without the tenderness and positive care given to him by Karen.

I hope this book will provide not only a wealth of knowledge and guidance but also provide inspiration to those who have cancer to continue fighting and to those loved ones who provide care.

—Marty

"Experience Is Not What Happens to You; It's What You Do with What Happens to You"

—Aldous Huxley

Dear Karen—Your overwhelming support and comfort have been more than a crutch these last five years. Watching your strength during Monty's illness and following Monty's death have been an inspiration to all those you encounter.

> Thank you and
> With much love forever,
> Your friend,
>
> —Roz

Dear Roz—What would I ever have done without you during this time? You were always there for me to share my experiences whether good or difficult. Your constant support was so special and helpful.

> With much love and friendship,
> —Karen

Source Acknowledgments

Adria Laboratories. *Cancer Terms*. Ed. Adria Laboratories. Columbus, OH, 1993.

American Association of Retired Persons. *A Path For Caregivers*. Washington, DC, 1996.

American Association of Retired Persons. *About Health Care Powers of Attorney and Living Wills*. Washington, DC, 1995.

American Association of Retired Persons. *Medicare: What It Covers, What It Doesn't*. Washington, DC, 1997.

American Association of Retired Persons. *Miles Away and Still Caregiving*. Ed. Health Advocacy Services. Washington, DC, 1994.

American Association of Retired Persons. *Staying At Home: A Guide to Long-Term Care and Housing*. Washington, DC, 1996.

American Association of Retired Persons. *The Family and Medical Leave Act*. Ed. Health Advocacy Services. Washington, DC, 1995.

American Cancer Society. *Americans With Disability Act: Legal Protection Against Employment Discrimination*. Ed. American Cancer Society. Washington, D.C., 1993.

American Cancer Society. *Cancer Word Book*. Ed. American Cancer Society. Washington, D.C., 1990.

American Cancer Society. *Caring for the Patient with Cancer-at Home-A Guide for Patients and Families*. Ed. American Cancer Society. Washington, DC, 1998.

Benjamin, Harold, Ph.D. *The Wellness Community, Guide to Fighting for Recovery from Cancer*. Ed. Jeremy P. Tarcher/Putnam, Penguin Inc. New York, NY. 1995.

Benjamin, Harold, Ph.D. *From Victim to Victor*. Ed. Dell Publishing, Bantam Doubleday Dell Publishing Group, Inc. New York, NY. 1987.

Brener, Anne. *Mourning and Mitzvah.* Ed. Jewish Lights. VT, 1995.

Brown, Jr., H. Jackson. *Life's Little Instruction Book.* Ed. Rutledge House Press. Nashville, TN, 1991.

Carter, Rosalynn and Golant, Susan. *Helping Yourself Help Others.* Ed. Random House. New York, NY, 1994.

CNA Insurance. *Guide to Health Insurance for People with Medicare.* Ed. National Association of Insurance Companies and U.S. Department of Health and Human Services. Chicago, IL, 1995.

Fearing, Alanna and O'Donnell-Tormey. *Helpbook. What to do if Cancer Strikes.* Ed. Cancer Research Institute. New York, NY, 1993.

Gerson Institute. *The Gerson Primer.* Ed. Gerson and Straus. Bonita, CA., 1996.

Haller, James. *What to Eat When You Don't Feel Like Eating.* Ed. Lancelot Press. Hantsport, Nova Scotia, 1994.

Kirk, Juanda Morrison. *Caregiving: A Money Management Workbook.* Ed. American Association of Retired Persons. Consumer Affairs. Washingon, DC, 1992.

Kubler-Ross, Elisabeth. *On Children And Death.* Ed. Collier Books, Macmillan Publishing. New York, NY, 1993.

Kubler-Ross, Elisabeth. *Questions and Answers on Death and Dying.* Ed. Collier Books, Macmillan Publishing. New York, NY, 1993.

Joyce, Marilyn. *5 Minutes to Health.* Ed. Joyce. Los Angeles, CA, 1995.

Katzin, Carolyn. *Nutrition Handbook. The Wellness Community.* Ed. Katzen. Los Angeles, CA, 1995.

Lansky, Bruce. *Familiarity Breeds Children.* Ed. Simon & Schuster. Deephaven, MN, 1994.

National Cancer Institute, National Institutes of Health. *Action Guide for Healthy Eating.* Silver Springs, MD, 1995.

National Cancer Institute, National Institutes of Health. *Advanced Cancer—Living Each Day.* Silver Springs, MD, 1992.

National Cancer Institute, National Institutes of Health. *Chemotherapy and You.* Silver Springs, MD, 1991.

National Cancer Institute, National Institutes of Health. *Eating Hints for Cancer Patients.* Silver Springs, MD, 1998.

National Cancer Institute, National Institutes of Health. *Facing Forward: A Guide for Cancer Survivors.* Silver Springs, MD, 1992.

National Cancer Institute, National Institutes of Health. *Radiation Therapy and You.* Silver Springs, MD, 1993.

National Cancer Institute, National Institutes of Health. *Taking Time: Support For People With Cancer And The People Who Care About Them.* Silver Springs, MD, 1992.

National Cancer Institute, National Institutes of Health. *The Immune System-How it Works.* Silver Springs, MD, 1996.

National Cancer Institute, National Institutes of Health. *When Cancer Recurs.* Silver Springs, MD, 1990.

National Coalition for Cancer Survivorship. *What Cancer Survivors Need to Know About Health Insurance.* Silver Springs, MD, 1995.

National Coalition for Cancer Survivorship. *When Someone in Your Family Has Cancer.* Silver Springs, MD, 1995.

National Coalition for Cancer Survivorship. *Working It Out: Your Employment Rights As a Cancer Survivor.* Silver Springs, MD, 1995.

National Hospice Organization. *About Hospice.* South Deerfield, MA, 1985.

Prevention Magazine. Rodale Press, Inc. October, 1997.

Sanker, Andrea. *Dying At Home.* Ed. Bantam Books, Bantam Doubleday Dell Publishing Group, Inc. New York, NY, 1995.

Social Security Administration. *Social Security-Understanding the Benefits.* Washington, DC, 1998.

Stella Maris Clinic. *Basic Protocol at Stella Maris Clinic. Wholistic Intervention.* Tijuana, BC, Mexico, 1997.

U.S. Department of Health and Human Services. *Medicare & You 2000.* Ed. Health Care Financing Administration. Washington, DC, 2000.

U.S. Department of Veterans Affairs. *Federal Benefits for Veterans and Dependents.* Ed. Office of Public Affairs. Washington, DC, 1998.

Permissions

We would like to acknowledge and thank the following
people for the permission to use their material:

H. Jackson Brown, Jr.

Judge Cohen

Pamela Elyse Sussman

Randy Glasbergen

Ted Goff

Index

"The book provides helpful tools to caregivers who can easily get overwhelmed during a time of need. Congratulations on such a powerful accomplishment."
                    —**Jacqueline Bell,** Chairwoman of the Board, Israel
                              Cancer Research Fund, Los Angeles Chapter

"This is an essential sourcebook and is accurate, detailed and highly practical...a treasure of information. Outstanding presentation. Exactly what families have lacked until now."
                    —**Catherine Klatzker**, RN, Pediatric ICU Children's
                              Hospital, Los Angeles

"A wonderful roadmap on cancer caregiving, encompassing invaluable information that will coach, mentor and navigate people through a difficult passage of life."
                    —**Dorothy L. Means**, LCSW, Oncology Health Care
                              Professional, Los Angeles

"Every cancer patient needs an advocate. This resource provides abundant hints and data that will make caregiving easier. A well-organized, practical, and personal guide."
                    —**Cheryl Hoffman, M.D.**, Section Chief-Cardiovascular
                              and Interventional Radiology, Los Alamitos
                              Hospital

"The ultimate message is to face the challenge, claim the spirit to fight this disease with just the right balance of advocacy, information, love and even humor. A useful guidebook that combines pragmatic advice with the sensitivity of personal experiences."
                    —**Antonette Krpan, D.C.**, Alternative Health Care
                              Provider, Los Angeles

"As a cancer survivor, your book would have been very helpful for us. Your book will help thousands of people better understand this dreaded disease and how to handle it."
                    —**Bobbye & Mort Steinberg**, Cancer Survivor/
                              Caregiver, Past Presidents, Stop Cancer

"Your guide is a treasure...a must read for caregivers. Page after page, your loving tribute is filled with valuable information."
                    —**Pat Harvey,** Cancer Caregiver, California KCAL-TV9,
                              News Anchor, Los Angeles

"A *must* on every caregiver's booklist. I wish I could have had this book to give every person who has ever come to The Wellness Community for support."
—**Sangeeta Levy, Ph.D.**, MFT, Group Facilitator/
Workshop Leader, The Wellness Community,
Santa Monica

"In these pages you will find treasures of insight and love to renew life and restore the spirit. You will also find a warm and caring fellowship from those who have found that life with cancer still has meaning, joy, and celebration."
—**Rabbi Edward M. Feinstein**, Cancer Survivor, Valley
Beth Shalom, Rabbi of the Year (1995),
Los Angeles

"I witnessed the loving care provided….this is a labor of love. The authors have found a way of using their difficult experiences to help others facing similar challenges. May their words bring you direction, comfort, and peace."
—**Rabbi Levi Meier, Ph.D.**, Chaplain, Cedars Sinai
Medical Center, Los Angeles

"A monumental contribution to the body of cancer literature. Hundreds of essential tips provide a unique resource for not only the caregiver, but also the patient, family and friends. I am anxious to recommend this book."
—**David George**, Executive Director, Stop Cancer,
Los Angeles